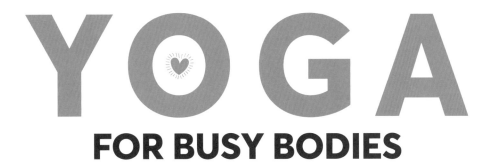

YOGA

FOR BUSY BODIES

JANET LEE

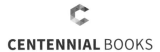

CENTENNIAL BOOKS

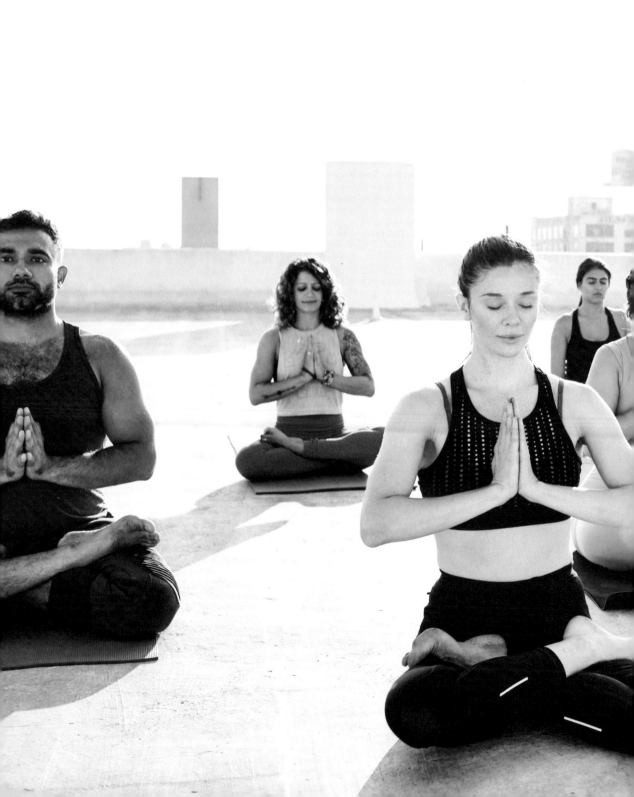

YOGA

FOR BUSY BODIES

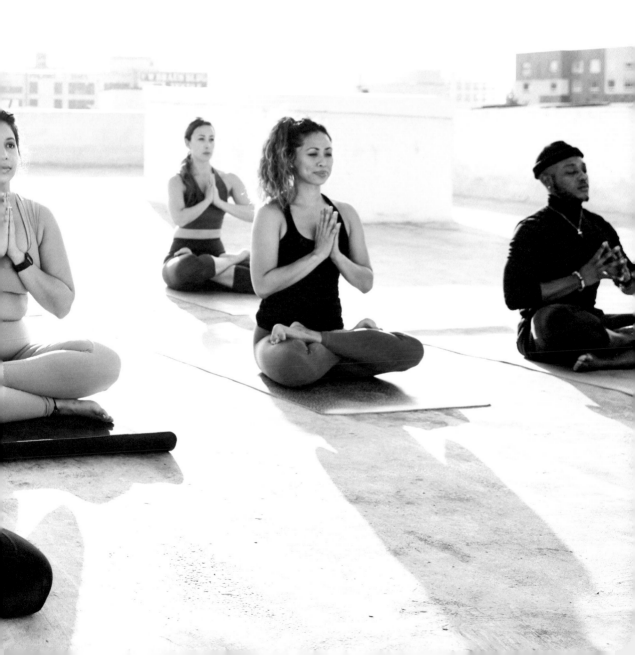

CONTENTS

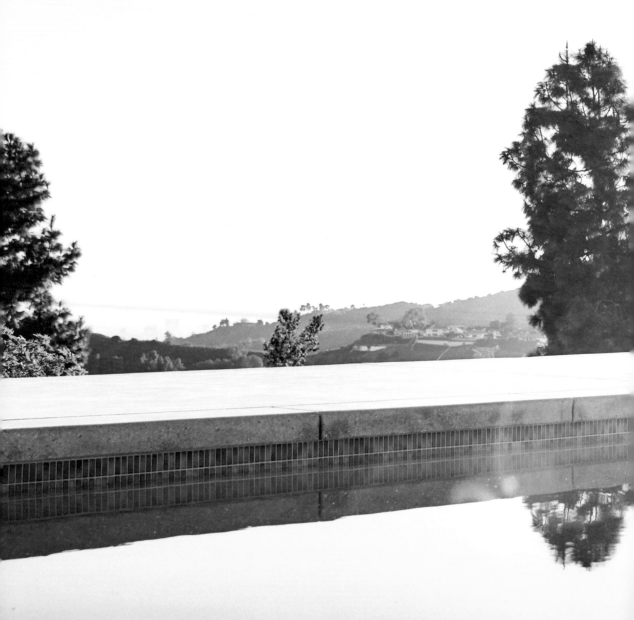

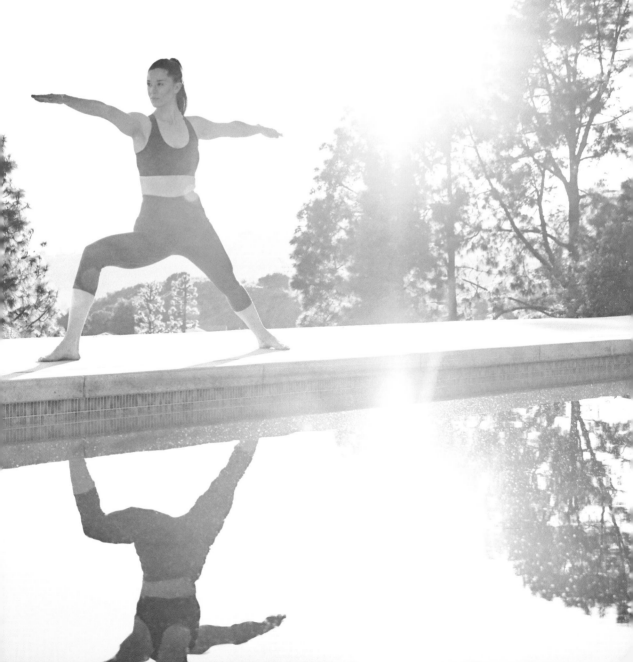

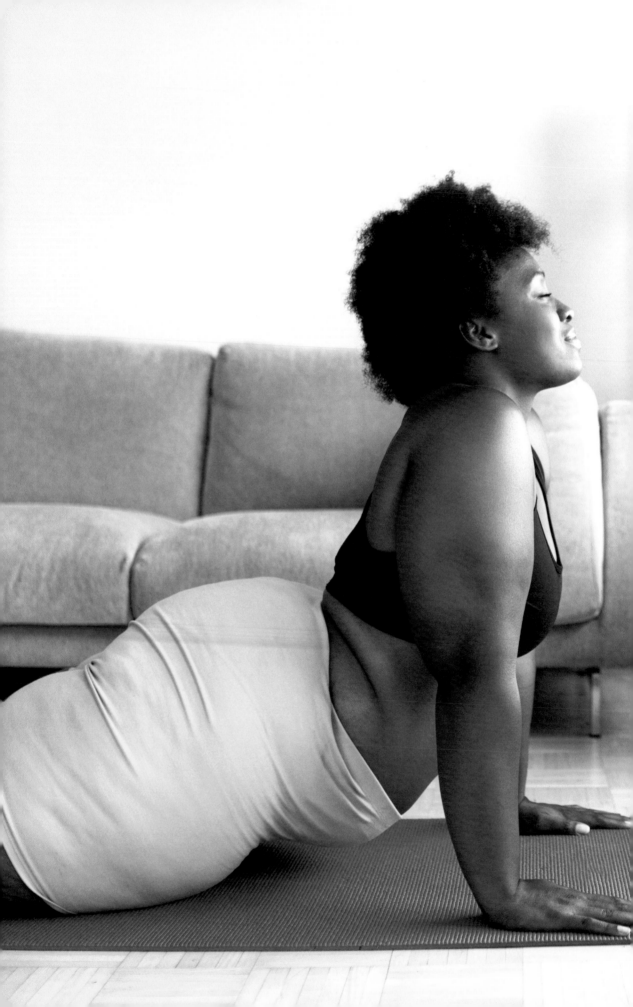

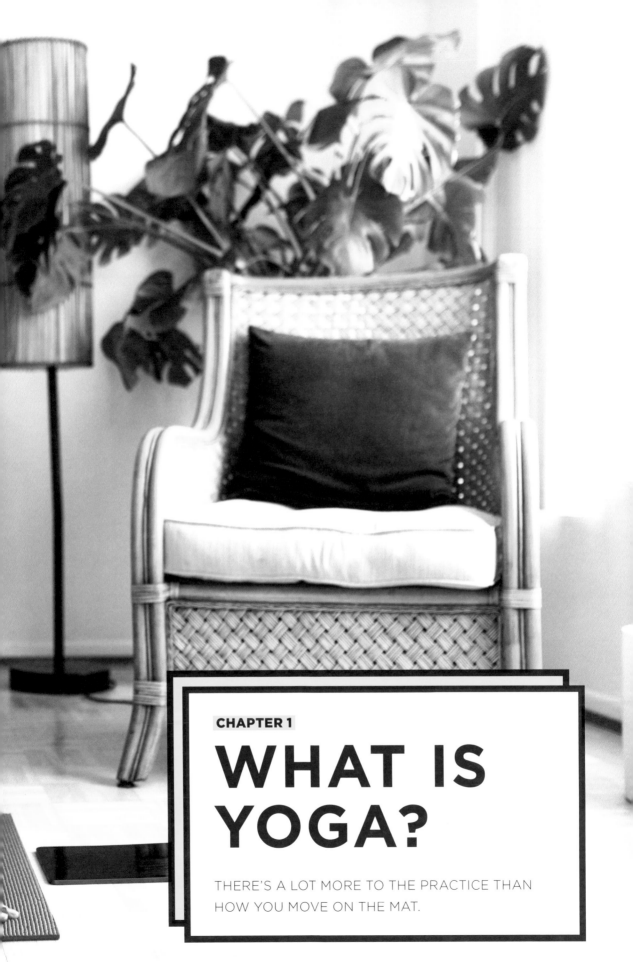

CHAPTER 1

WHAT IS YOGA?

THERE'S A LOT MORE TO THE PRACTICE THAN HOW YOU MOVE ON THE MAT.

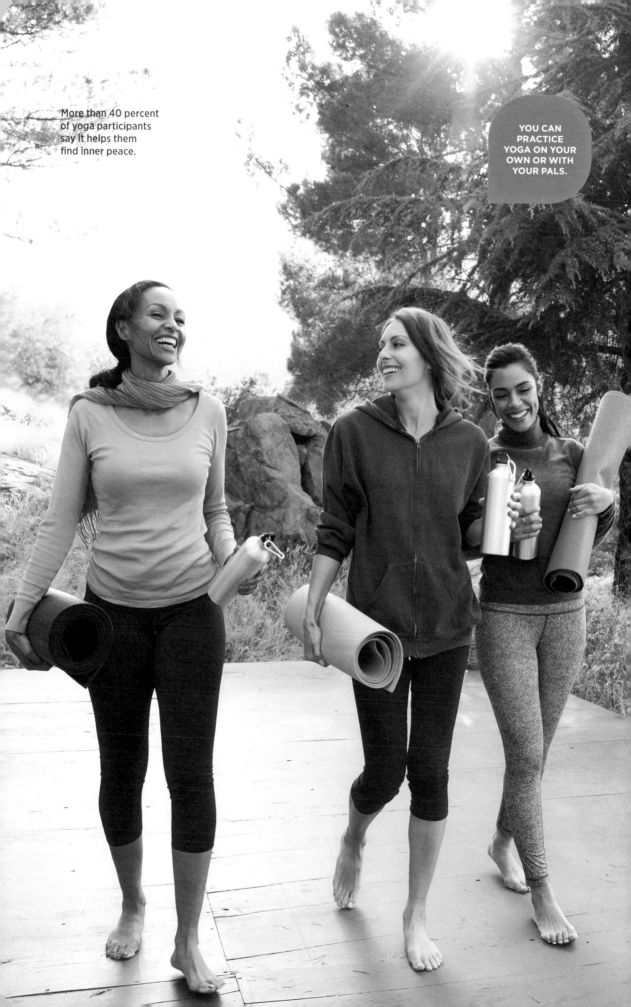

More than 40 percent of yoga participants say it helps them find inner peace.

YOU CAN PRACTICE YOGA ON YOUR OWN OR WITH YOUR PALS.

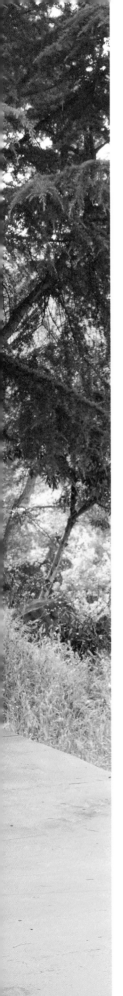

WELCOME TO THE YOGA LIFESTYLE

THIS POPULAR WORKOUT-SLASH-WAY-OF-LIVING HAS GONE MAINSTREAM, ATTRACTING FANS AND BUSINESS OPPORTUNITIES AROUND THE GLOBE. HERE'S A CLOSER LOOK AT YOGA TODAY —AND BACK IN THE DAY.

What was once created as a way to achieve a sort of oneness of mind, body and spirit while living with compassion, integrity and generosity has morphed into something entirely different. Close to 40 million people practice yoga in the United States, according to a study released by Yoga Alliance and *Yoga Journal*. It's in gyms across the country; there are studios for all types of yoga (hot, power, Ashtanga, Kundalini); and "corporate" chain yoga centers, such as CorePower Yoga, are spreading as well. Kids are doing it at school and universities are studying the many health benefits, from treating back pain to addiction.

The yoga "lifestyle" has spread off the mat too. Yogis spend more than $16 billion annually on accessories, especially clothing. In fact, those figure-flattering pieces spawned their own booming

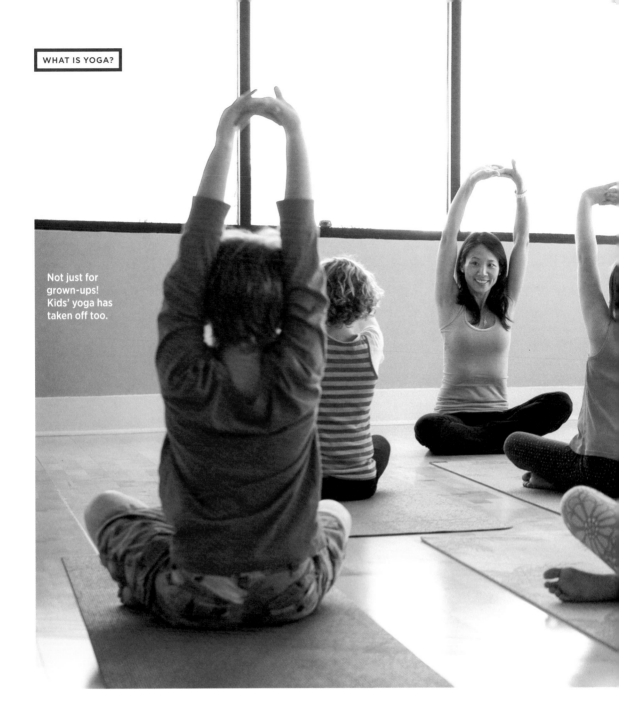

Not just for grown-ups! Kids' yoga has taken off too.

fashion category: athleisure. The "yoga diet"—heavy on green juice and veggies and light on meat, gluten and processed foods—has sparked a revolution in how we view clean eating as well. Even meditation, an important part of the bigger yoga picture, is going mainstream. It's a multibillion-dollar industry on its own, with studios opening around the country and tons of apps to help you drop in and get centered no matter where you are.

As with virtually every aspect of modern life, it's also been tainted by scandal. Big-name teachers have taken advantage of their positions and as a result, yoga has found itself in the middle of the #MeToo movement (and at the forefront of the push for more inclusivity).

Then there's social media. It may have done more than anything else to spread the word about the benefits of yoga and what the yoga lifestyle looks like, albeit somewhat one-dimensionally.

Whatever brings you to yoga, you get out of it what you put in. It will meet you where you are and show you a way to a better you. To truly experience everything that is yoga, though, you need to delve into the original philosophy of the practice.

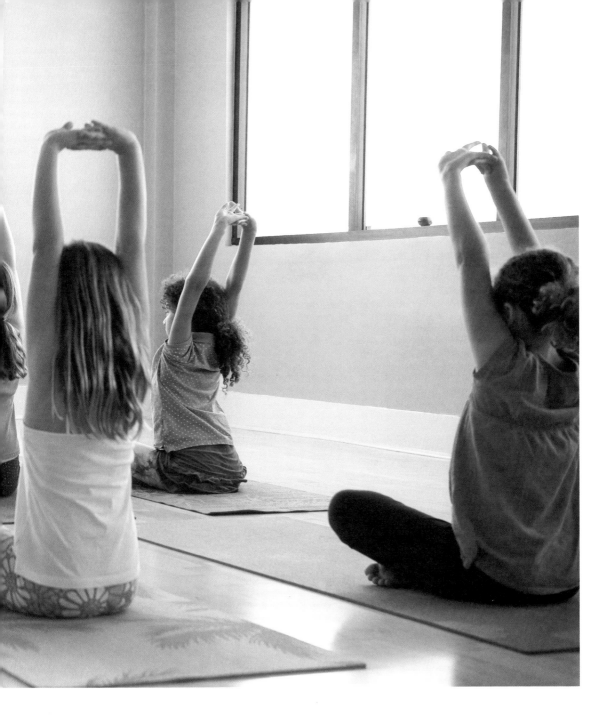

THE YOGIC PATH

What most people think of as yoga—the poses and stretches you do in a regular class—is only one aspect of a much larger picture. In fact, the poses, or asanas, are a fairly modern addition to the traditional yoga practice and philosophy. (The word asana means "seat" in Sanskrit.) Originally, yoga was purely a mental and philosophical pursuit.

A teacher, or guru, would answer questions from students—who were all men, by the way—about the meaning of life and teach them to meditate silently for hours on end to achieve inner peace. The students did simple poses beforehand to prepare their bodies for these long philosophical discussions and meditation while seated on an unforgiving floor. Today's yoga teachers add their knowledge of biomechanics, anatomy and the nervous system to teach classes that encourage holistic well-being and, above all, a strong, undistracted connection of mind, body and spirit in the present moment.

The word "yoga" loosely translates as "to yoke" or "to join together in union." "Yoga means connection between the individual's outer consciousness with the inner self," says Nicolai Bachman, author of *The Path of the Yoga Sutras*. This connection leads to a feeling of overall peace and ease.

Many studios will teach yoga as a lifestyle, including the eight-limbed path (see below), but it's hard to fit thousands of years of philosophy into a single class. There's a reason yoga is considered a practice. It's something you revisit on deepening levels of action and awareness day after day.

Part of the appeal of yoga is in finding stillness even in a chaotic world.

THE EIGHT LIMBS

Yamas Five universal guidelines for living with others in your community

Niyamas Five personal practices that can help you achieve a healthy, balanced life

Asanas Postures that strengthen your muscles and relieve pain in your physical body to prepare it for seated meditation

Pranayama Breathing practices that harness prana, your innate life force

Pratyahara Drawing your physical senses inward to reduce distractions and improve focus

Dharana Developing strong, mindful concentration on one thing

Dhyana The ability to calmly abide in the present moment through uninterrupted meditation

Samadhi Total inner peace; the bliss of experiencing integration of mind, body, spirit; what all yogis strive for

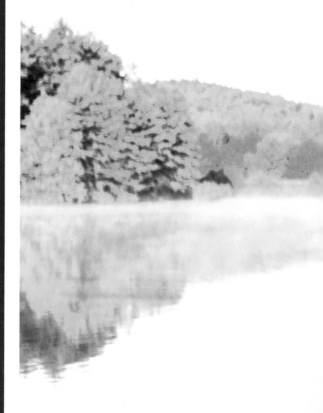

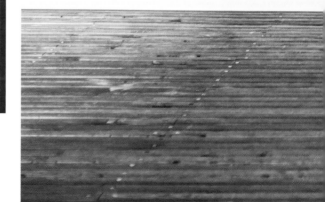

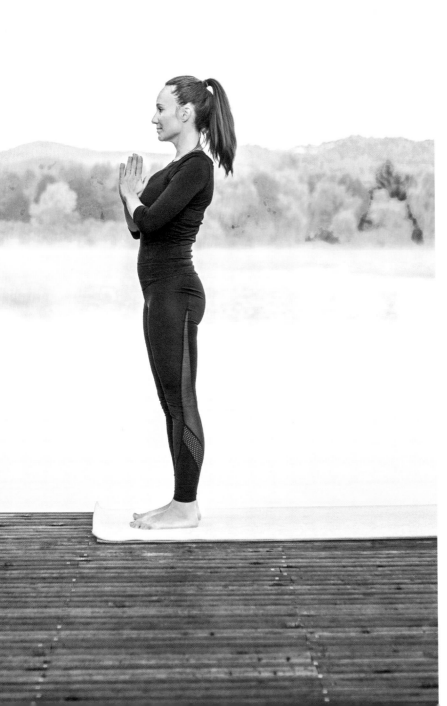

BY THE BOOK

The foundational text of yoga is the *Yoga Sutras of Patanjali*, a small book of nearly indecipherable "threads" of knowledge written between 200 BC and 200 AD in ancient Sanskrit. (Compare "sutra" to the English word "suture," or stitch.) These short threads of wisdom, written by a teacher named Patanjali, tell us that yoga is the practice of consciously directing our thoughts inward, away from external chaos. Patanjali wrote, "Yoga is the cessation of the fluctuation of the waves of thoughts that distort peace in the heart and mind."

The way to do this is through the "eight-limbed path of classical yoga" (see box, left) that anyone can incorporate into their own life. "It consists of practices that refine and stabilize your body, breath and mind for the purpose of cultivating inner happiness," explains instructor Nicolai Bachman. "Yoga is a way of life that contributes to a happy, civil, caring society."

13

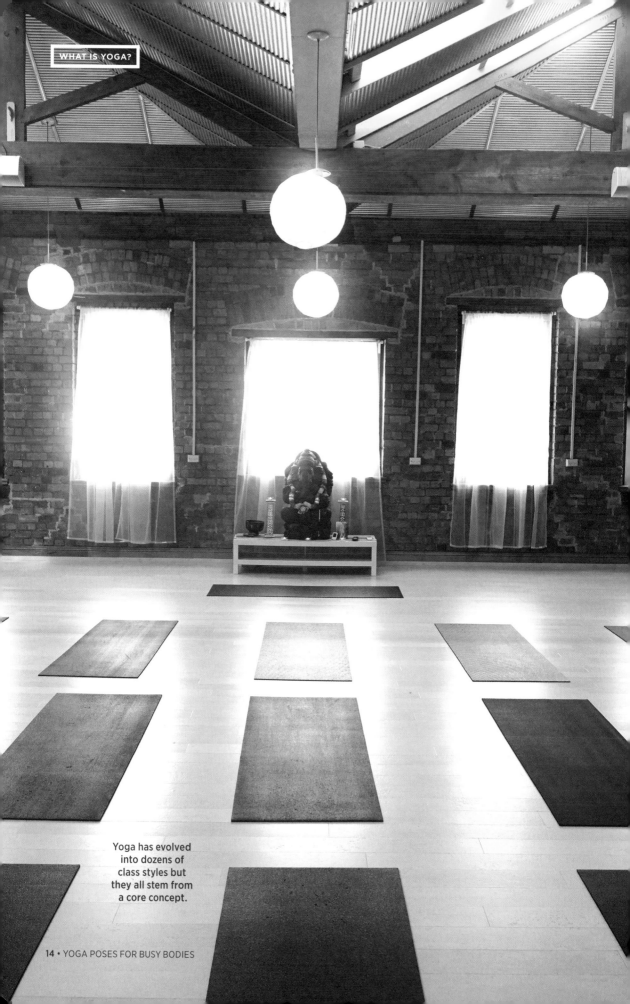

Yoga has evolved into dozens of class styles but they all stem from a core concept.

THE YAMAS AND NIYAMAS

You don't have to master one limb before going on to another. You can integrate all of these concepts even in one yoga practice (think: focusing on breathing, concentrating on balance and staying present in a pose). The interesting thing is that the first two limbs—the yamas and niyamas—basically provide a "do's and don'ts" list for life off the yoga mat, so they're an easy place to start.

YAMAS

These are actions (often requiring some self-control) that reduce the opportunity for conflict in your community, whether that's with your family, friends, neighbors or colleagues. They include:

AHIMSA Showing compassion to all beings (including yourself) through actions and thoughts steeped in the philosophy of non-harming and non-violence.

ASTEYA Being trustworthy and not stealing others' thoughts, energy or possessions.

SATYA Living with integrity and speaking with truthfulness. Saying what you mean and meaning what you say.

BRAHMACHARYA Living a balanced lifestyle—not working 24/7 or partying all the time—so that you have time and energy to pursue spiritual maturity.

APARIGRAHA Living generously and within your means and sharing with others.

NIYAMAS

These are primarily inwardly focused practices that cultivate a healthy mind and healthy body.

SAUCHA Purity of thought and actions of self-love. Being mindful of what information you consume (news, Twitter) so your mind doesn't get overly cluttered. Taking care of your possessions; clearing out your house to reduce negative energy. Caring for your body so that you stay healthy and strong.

SANTOSHA Striving to stay present to experience joy right now instead of living anxiously in the future.

TAPAS Dedication and enthusiasm for yoga practice and life in general. It's the zest for life that gets you out of bed and onto the yoga mat each day.

SVADHYAYA Study of inspirational texts outside of yoga class—taking a course in Buddhism, studying with your rabbi or reading poetry, for example.

ISHVARA-PRANIDHANA Surrender and devotion to a higher power. Ishvara is typically considered to be a universal, shared wisdom that all humans have access to. This niyama inspires humility—we don't know it all—and the sharing of ideas between individuals and cultures.

THE SIX BRANCHES OF YOGA

HOW DO YOU YOGA?

The ultimate goal of yoga is the concept of union, but like any journey, there are different paths, called "margas," to get there, says Diane Finlayson, chair of the yoga therapy department at Maryland University of Integrative Health.

BHAKTI YOGA is about devotion to "God" and seeing that divinity in everything that's around you.

HATHA YOGA uses movement to work the physical body.

JNANA YOGA is a more intellectual approach that involves digging deep into scripture and other yogic texts and studying all aspects of yoga.

KARMA YOGA focuses on selfless service, such as volunteering and giving back to the community, with no expectation of getting "credit" for it.

RAJA YOGA emphasizes meditation and contemplation, with special attention on the eight limbs.

TANTRIC YOGA utilizes rituals and reverence—it's not all about sex—to celebrate the divine.

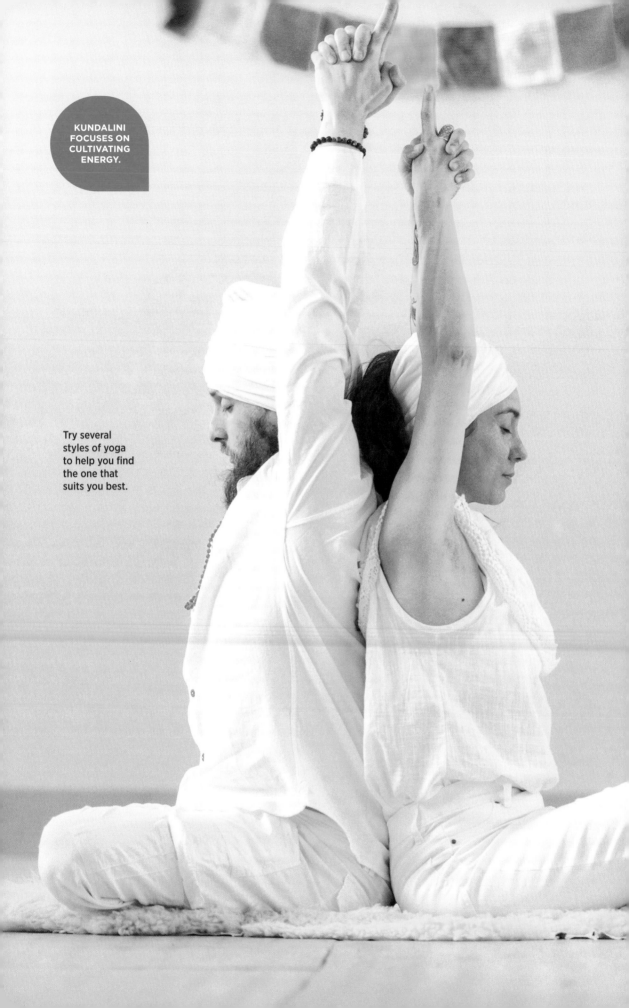

KUNDALINI FOCUSES ON CULTIVATING ENERGY.

Try several styles of yoga to help you find the one that suits you best.

WHAT'S IN A NAME?

IN YOGA, FINDING THE RIGHT STYLE AND PRACTICE IS A PROCESS OF EXPERIMENTATION. THERE ARE MANY KINDS TO CONSIDER—SO DON'T LIMIT YOURSELF.

One of the potentially confusing things when starting down the yoga path is figuring out which style to take. Ashtanga or Iyengar? Gentle or hot? Is there a difference?

"Krishnamacharya was the one who started the Hatha style of yoga back in the late 1800s and early 1900s," says Diane Finlayson, E-RYT, chair of the yoga therapy department at Maryland University of Integrative Health in Baltimore. "He used to have students give yoga gymnastics demonstrations, and it's thought that out of those, the British became interested in yoga for health. That was the beginning of group-style yoga classes. Now, it's what you see in gyms and studios all over the place." Over time, while the basic poses, or asanas, have stayed much the same, different teachers have taken those exercises and formed their own approaches.

The asana-focused yoga that most people are familiar with is known as Hatha Yoga. "It's a series of postures that work the body," says Finlayson. Ashtanga, Iyengar, hot, power, restorative and Anusara Yoga are all Hatha styles. Some classes may be more focused on movement, while others are centered around alignment or holding postures.

While Hatha is an overarching term, it can also be used to refer to a class that includes a gentler approach and more held postures versus faster flows.

Those flowing classes are known as Vinyasa-style yoga, which is also considered Hatha. In it, you flow quickly from pose to pose, pairing the breath with each movement and building heat. A "vinyasa" can also refer to a Sun Salutation sequence that might be incorporated between poses to increase body heat and link moves together.

The styles below are the main types of classes you'll see on a schedule. If you really want to dive into a particular practice, find a studio that's devoted to a single style, such as Kundalini or Ashtanga.

ANUSARA "It's kind of the kinder, gentler Iyengar," says Finlayson. "It works with accessing the flow of energy in the body while still including a focus on alignment and breathwork." It also has a strong spiritual bent. Teachers provide heart-centered themes for each class, such as recognizing your own goodness and the goodness in others.

ASHTANGA A flowing, fast-paced, athletic class that involves a set sequence of asanas divided into six series, Ashtanga Yoga was created by Sri K. Pattabhi Jois. "Sometimes it gets a reputation for being really strict and disciplined, so people are intimidated by it, especially beginners," says Kristen Stanley, E-RYT, a yoga teacher at Steadfast & True Yoga in Nashville, Tennessee. "I believe there's an opening for anyone to start wherever they are. It's really designed to be more of a personal practice."

HOT YOGA This style, done in a room heated to 105 degrees or warmer, is a go-to for anyone who enjoys the physical and mental challenge of pushing through the heat. Many people, especially athletes, appreciate the flexibility boost the temps give their tight muscles.

IYENGAR Founded by B.K.S. Iyengar, this type of Hatha Yoga is very focused on alignment—making sure your arms, legs and joints are doing exactly what they're supposed to do in each pose to minimize injury. "If you have some structural issues, like shoulder or knee problems, seek out an Iyengar class," says Finlayson.

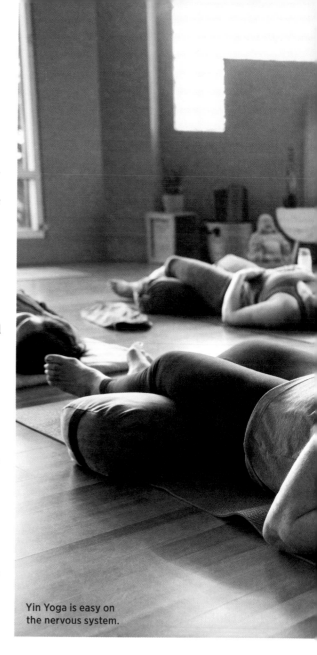
Yin Yoga is easy on the nervous system.

KUNDALINI Practitioners here focus on the breath and energy systems of the body versus structure. Although some of the poses are similar to Hatha yoga, it's not a Hatha style. Kundalini was created by Yogi Bhajan, who combined the poses with breathing and mantras and used them for various purposes, such as to help energize the body, boost digestion or reduce headaches.

POWER YOGA An offshoot of Ashtanga Yoga—without the rigidity—power yoga is all about vinyasa: flowing, athletic asanas. There are many different styles of power yoga, depending on the

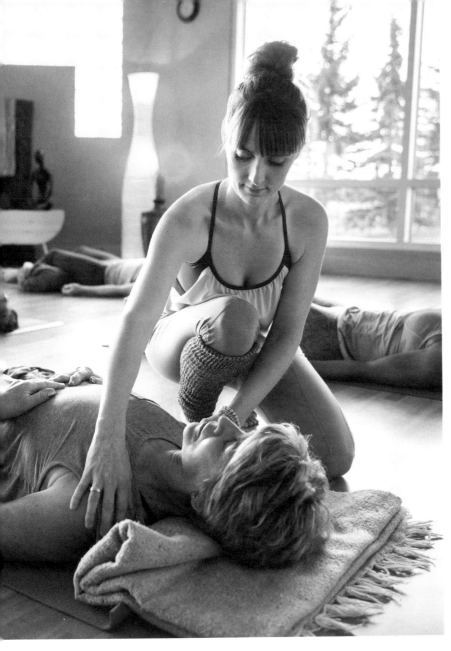

WHAT IS YOGA THERAPY?

Considering the many health benefits of yoga—research has shown it helps treat depression, high blood pressure, back pain, headaches and more—there's an opportunity to bring yoga into the medical setting, as therapy, to work with a variety of populations.

A yoga therapist is to yoga what a personal trainer is to fitness. If you want a personal prescription to get stronger or fitter, you see a trainer. And if you have a specific health goal, or maybe you have scoliosis or a torn labrum, you want to work with someone who can adjust your form and recommend individualized poses to help. "A yoga therapist will work with you to create a set of practices—including meditation, asanas and breathing—that will help you get well," says Maryland University of Integrative Health's Diane Finlayson. Yoga therapists are certified from the International Association of Yoga Therapists. Go to iayt .org for more info.

teacher. If you're looking for a yoga class to raise your heart rate and get a "workout," this will do it.

YIN The antithesis of power ("yang") yoga, Yin is all about holding stretches and targeting the connective tissue around joints. It's sometimes referred to as gentle or restorative yoga, but make no mistake: There is physical work being done. The long holds (several minutes) can be uncomfortable, but create an opportunity to practice patience and sit with the emotions that arise. If the idea of being still for so long makes you anxious, it's probably a sign you should give it a try. (For more, see page 136).

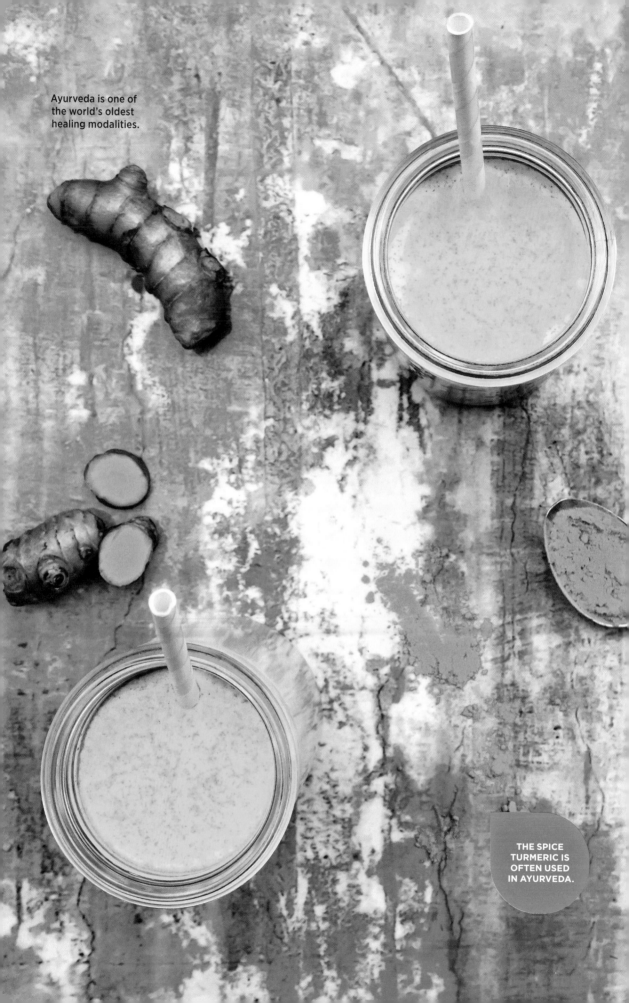

Ayurveda is one of the world's oldest healing modalities.

THE SPICE TURMERIC IS OFTEN USED IN AYURVEDA.

AT-HOME HEALING

AYURVEDA, A TRADITIONAL HEALING SCIENCE THAT ORIGINATED IN INDIA, CAN COMPLEMENT YOUR YOGA PRACTICE AND ENHANCE YOUR HEALTH AND LIFE.

We're lucky to be alive in a time when there's so much information at our fingertips, whether it's about a random trivia question or a health concern (paging Dr. Google!). When it comes to those health issues, there's a system of medicine that says this information—what's best for your body—has always been at our fingertips. We just have to take the time to look up from our devices and tune in to nature. The system is Ayurveda, and it's one of the oldest sustained forms of medicine on the planet.

Known as the science of life and the sister science of yoga, Ayurveda is rooted in India and dates back about 5,000 years. Whereas yoga is considered a study of the mind that also uses the body as a tool (through postures, or asanas), Ayurveda is a study of the body that says complete health includes both body and mind. And while yoga is like Ayurveda's spiritual system, Ayurveda can be considered yoga's medical system, keeping you healthy while you pursue your path toward self-realization.

As a means for healing, Ayurveda integrates yogic practices such as asanas, pranayama (breathing exercises) and meditation. It also uses self-reflection

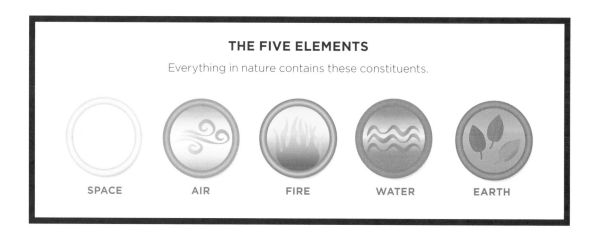

THE FIVE ELEMENTS

Everything in nature contains these constituents.

SPACE AIR FIRE WATER EARTH

as a way to pursue a clear, sound mind, which practitioners believe is integral to overall good health. While the two systems are interrelated, it's not essential that you study yoga and Ayurveda together. Each is born from a rich philosophy and tradition that allows it to stand on its own.

Though it might be easy to deem Ayurveda outdated—especially given Western medicine's many advances and cures for diseases—Eastern medicine has an important and harmonious role to play in our modern world. While Western medicine excels at helping us cure deeply rooted diseases and heal from acute trauma, Ayurveda finds its strong suit in health maintenance and the prevention of disease. It offers comprehensive recommendations for daily and seasonal routines with the aim of supporting an individual's specific needs.

WHAT'S YOUR CONSTITUTION?

Ayurveda can be classified as a "natural" medicine thanks to its therapeutic use of plants versus pharmaceuticals, and because it takes into account that we, too, are a part of nature. Its foundational principle, called the "macrocosm-microcosm continuum," suggests that each of us is a mini replica of nature or the universe. When nature undergoes a shift, we also feel a change internally. Likewise, our actions will also impact nature in some way.

Nature is comprised of five elements: ether (or space), air, fire, water and earth. These five elements are found in everything and everyone, and are necessary for the survival of all living things: We need space to move and expand, air to breathe, fire to process and transform, water to drink and earth to find our roots and grow.

Each season, plant, animal and person has its own unique expression of these elements. For example, an aloe plant, a chili pepper and a maple tree arguably need each of the five elements to thrive, but an aloe plant contains more water, a chili pepper has more fire and a maple tree has more earth. People are no different. We need all of the elements to survive, but a varying expression of each of the elements causes us to look different, have our own strengths and weaknesses and possess a unique set of personality traits and characteristics. You likely know people who are cool and watery like aloe, fiery like a pepper or grounded like a tree. Though each person may have things in common, our specific needs and interests will vary because of this unique elemental makeup. This is true even when it comes to yoga. For example, fiery people may gravitate toward a practice that has more strengthening qualities and structure, like in Ashtanga Yoga, whereas watery or earthy people could be drawn to a Yin Yoga practice.

These unique constitutions are known as doshas. A dosha is a combination of two elements and it governs specific systems and functions of the body and mind. Each of us contains all of the doshas to varying degrees, but typically one is dominant.

Vata dosha is a combination of ether and air and presides over movement, the nervous system, elimination, communication and creativity.

Pitta dosha is made of fire and water and oversees all things that transform, such as digestive fire and hormones, and also plays a key role in the ability to focus and have mental sharpness.

Kapha dosha is a blend of water and earth and contributes to immunity, growth and stability, along with the ability to be compassionate and nurturing beings.

Through the Ayurvedic lens, every individual has his or her own special doshic makeup, called your *prakriti*. Your ideal diet and lifestyle is determined by your prakriti. Maintaining these healthy practices will help you thrive and stay well. When an element or dosha starts to accumulate beyond your original state—perhaps due to unhealthy lifestyle choices—you may begin to feel unwell. This is a doshic imbalance, or *vikriti*. Any element or dosha can get out of balance, but it's your dominant one that typically causes problems.

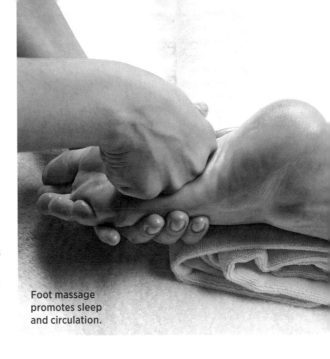

Foot massage promotes sleep and circulation.

PUT IT TO USE

Ayurveda can be applied to your life in a range of ways, from how you start your day to your ideal career. You can easily weave some practices into your routine, no matter what your prakriti.
1 Drink warm water in the morning to increase your ability to digest food.
2 Use a tongue cleaner to enhance your ability to taste food.
3 Dry-brush your body to boost circulation.
4 Make lunch your biggest meal, since your body digests the best between 10 a.m. and 2 p.m.
5 Apply oil to your feet at night, a calming (and meditative) practice that can promote better sleep.

When you do come down with a cold, acne or indigestion, or have a poor night's sleep—signs of a vikriti—medicinal spices and herbal remedies (turmeric, ginger, cardamom, ashwagandha, shatavari or brahmi), breathing practices and even specific bodywork can help. Finally, if you experience traumatic injury, more chronic conditions, or those that are deeply manifested—such as rheumatoid arthritis, autoimmune disorders or cancer—Ayurveda can serve as a complementary form of care, helping to lay a foundation of health and to increase the effectiveness of other treatments

FIRST, DO YOUR RESEARCH.

FINDING AN AYURVEDA PRACTITIONER

You have to do a little homework when looking for an Ayurvedic professional. There is no national licensing body for Ayurveda in the U.S., but the National Ayurvedic Medical Association (NAMA), founded in 1998, has established criteria for three different levels of providers. (Go to ayurvedanama.org to find a practitioner.) **AYURVEDIC HEALTH COUNSELORS (AHC)** receive at least 600 hours of education and are qualified to provide support for health maintenance and disease prevention through dietary and lifestyle recommendations. **CERTIFIED AYURVEDIC PRACTITIONERS (CAP)** receive a minimum of 1,500 hours of education and are clinically trained to assist in disease management. They work with therapeutic herbs, in addition to health promotion. **AYURVEDIC DOCTORS (AD)** have graduated from a five-and-a-half year Bachelors of Ayurvedic Medicine and Surgery (BAMS) program in India and have the most extensive scope of practice.

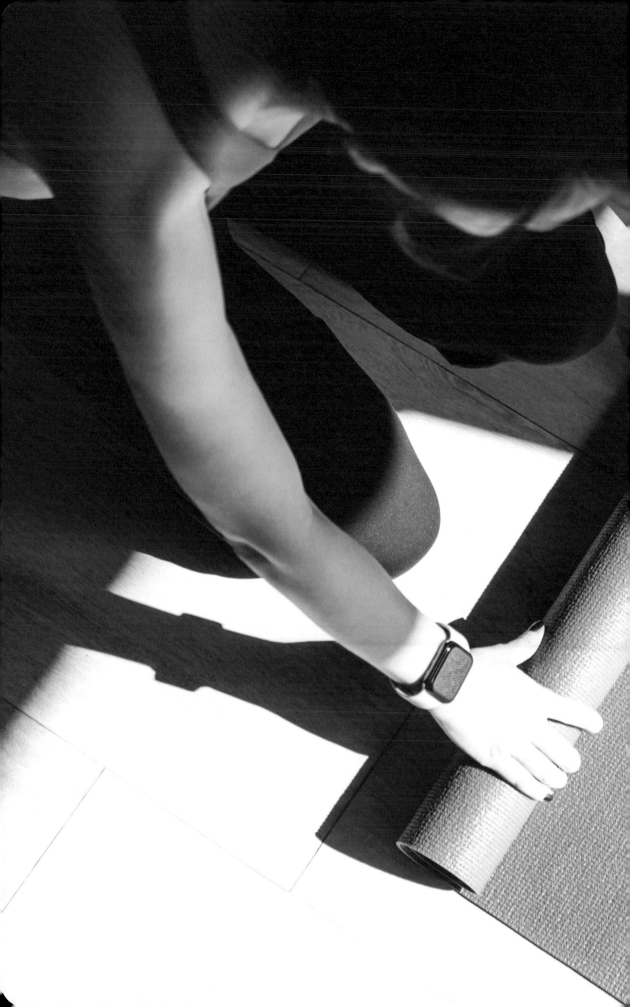

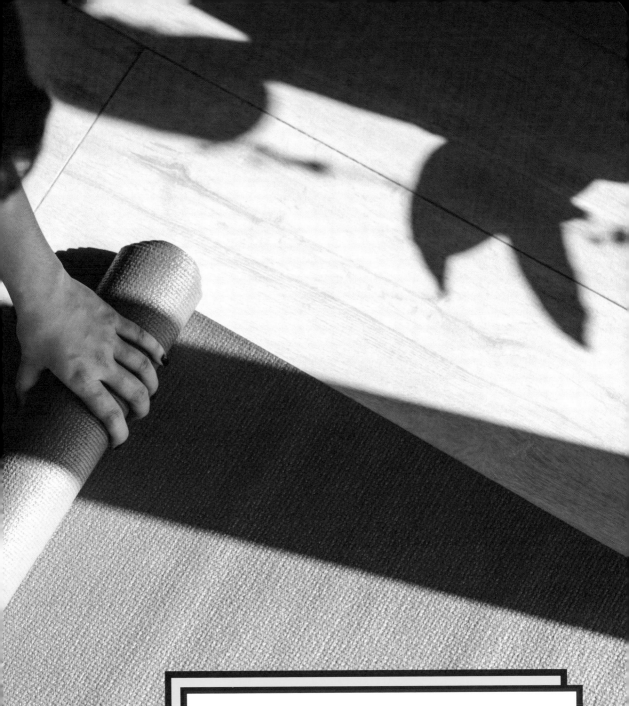

CHAPTER 2

A NEW START

YOGA MAKES YOU FEEL STRONG AND CENTERED—EVEN BEYOND THE PHYSICAL POSES.

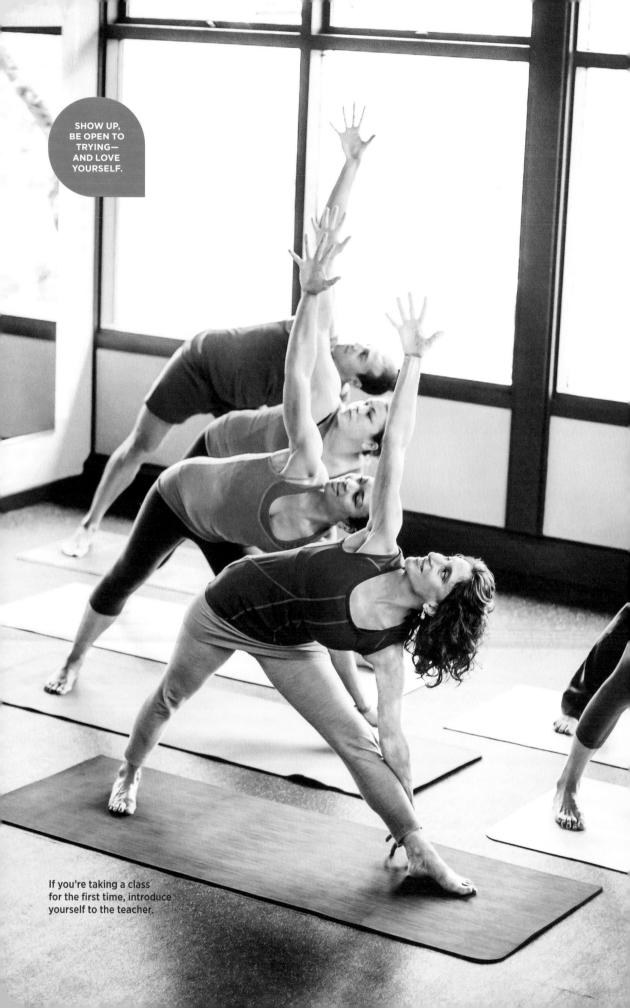

SHOW UP,
BE OPEN TO
TRYING—
AND LOVE
YOURSELF.

If you're taking a class
for the first time, introduce
yourself to the teacher.

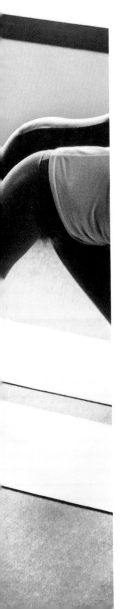

YOGA 101

FROM GEAR TO GARB TO WHAT TO EXPECT IN YOUR FIRST CLASS. OUR BEGINNER-FRIENDLY PRIMER WILL HAVE YOU CRAVING MORE MAT TIME IN NO TIME.

I f you're a social media fan, you may *think* you know what yoga's all about: super-bendy people doing spine-swiveling poses on gorgeous beaches. Or maybe you've heard rumors of those hot yoga classes where students emerge looking like they just ran a 10K in a tropical jungle. Regardless, it's easy to see why yoga—from the outside—may seem a little intimidating, like an exclusive club you don't have a key to. But that couldn't be further from the truth.

Yoga adapts to everybody and every *body*. Whether you're feeling like you're too tight, too weak or too heavy, yoga will meet you there, says Kali Om, E-RYT, a yoga instructor in Chicago and author of *Beyond the Mat: Don't Just Do Yoga—Live It*. "It's the perfect antidote to all those things. The beginner version of a pose gives you similar benefits to the advanced variation, and if you stick with it, your mind will be blown over and over again by what you're capable of."

So what's stopping you? Virtually every community has at least one place to do yoga, whether it's a gym, a private studio or a recreation center—and of course, we've got lots of great ways for you to start on the pages ahead. You don't even need shoes! "Yoga will give you radiant health and have a positive effect on every single part of your body, not just your musculoskeletal system," says Om. "But the impact it has on the mind—your ability to cultivate that single-pointed focus—is profound." In fact, many longtime practitioners consider their mat a refuge. The moment they step onto it, stress subsides, confidence flows in—and they feel like they're home.

Read on to learn everything you need to get started so you can experience what this extremely personal practice has to offer—and find your own piece of home wherever you are.

FIND A CLASS

Learning the basic poses firsthand and under a teacher's watchful eye can help make sure you are getting the movements right so you don't get injured or overdo it. "Try a few different teachers and styles," says San Francisco yoga instructor Jason Crandell, E-RYT. "A lot of what determines your experience in class is whether you resonate with the personality and approach of the teacher." If you don't like the first teacher you have, try again with someone else. When searching for your first class, look for a beginner or "Level 1" session on the schedule (see "The Yoga Code," right, for a breakdown of class ratings).

If it's your first time, get to class early and introduce yourself. If you're still not sure it's the right spot for you, go by the studio when there's no class and chat with the instructors. Ask about the types of yoga they offer and the instructors' training. States don't require certification or licensing, but many of today's yoga teacher-training programs have similar requirements. The minimum for many programs is 200 hours, with additional certification levels at 500, 800 and 1,000 hours. That means people who finish these trainings have put in at least that many hours studying to become a teacher or taking additional education to increase their knowledge.

In addition, instructors may have the credentials RYT or E-RYT after their names, a designation that is bestowed by the Yoga Alliance, a nonprofit advocacy group for the yoga profession that also sets standards for training. The credentials mean the instructor's training has met a certain minimum level of adequacy, usually 200 hours of teacher training. The "E" before RYT means the teacher has significant experience teaching, beyond their training.

"It's fairly rare now that studios will hire someone who doesn't have a 200-hour RYT certification," says Crandell. While the letters are meant to give you a sense of comfort about a teacher's experience, it's no guarantee they'll be good. Similarly, instructors who've been teaching for years may have trained in an apprentice- or mentor-type situation and may not have a certification sanctioned by Yoga Alliance. Regardless, the instructor should be happy to explain his or her background and training and allow you to decide for yourself by taking a class.

WHAT TO EXPECT

Each yoga class is different, but they tend to have similar structures. Classes last from 60 to 90 minutes, and you'll usually start with a quick meditation or some gentle poses to help you bring

---

THE YOGA CODE

Level 1 A slower-paced, beginner-level class that introduces breathing technique, basic postures and alignment.

Level 2 This will be a little faster paced , with an expectation that you know how to pair your movement with your breath and are familiar with many poses. You may be introduced to some advanced postures (including binds, balance poses and inversions) in this class, but you don't have to do them.

Level 3 This is an advanced class , often fast-paced, with more involved postures and less instruction on alignment. Regardless, always go at your own pace, especially if you have an injury or other limitation.

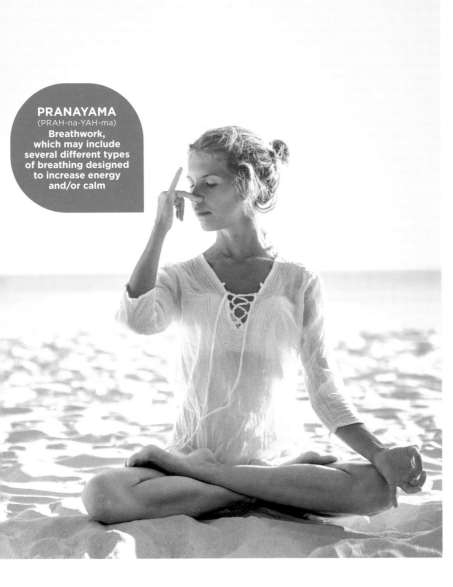

PRANAYAMA
(PRAH-na-YAH-ma)
Breathwork,
which may include
several different types
of breathing designed
to increase energy
and/or calm

Q What do I do if I'm not comfortable with the instructor touching me during a class?

A It's common for yoga teachers to give physical adjustments—to deepen your stretch or improve your alignment—but more people are opting out of them. "Your teacher may ask at the beginning of class if anyone prefers not to be adjusted, or they may use cards that you put at the front of the mat if you're passing," says San Francisco-based yoga instructor Jason Crandell. "Often, teachers will ask permission before they adjust you, or you can tell your teacher at the beginning of class."

THE NO. 1 THING TO KNOW!

IT'S ALL ABOUT THE BREATH

More important than the poses in yoga is your breathing. "The movement in yoga is all in service of the breath," says instructor Jason Crandell. "Regular, rhythmic breathing helps regulate the nervous system, which facilitates attention and relaxation." In a flowing class, you'll often be pairing a movement with the breath (bend forward as you exhale, straighten the spine as you inhale, for instance), while at other times you'll be breathing while you maintain a pose. You're never holding your breath, unless it's part of a specific exercise.

The typical style of breathing in yoga class is called *ujjayi* (oo-JAH-yee) breath. To do it, inhale and exhale through your nose, feeling your exhale "scraping" the back of your throat slightly. (If you were exhaling with your mouth open it would sound like you were saying "*haaaaa.*") This stimulates the vagus nerve, which enhances your ability to handle stress.

Q Can I ask questions in class if I'm confused?

A If it's something really important, try to get your teacher's attention. Otherwise, wait until the end and talk to your instructor afterward, says Chicago-based yoga instructor Kali Om. "Asking a question in class can be distracting for the flow," says Om. "That's why it's best to start with a beginner class, since the pace will be slower and there will be more explanation and coaching than in a higher-level session." If you're struggling with alignment, your teacher is likely to notice and come over to help.

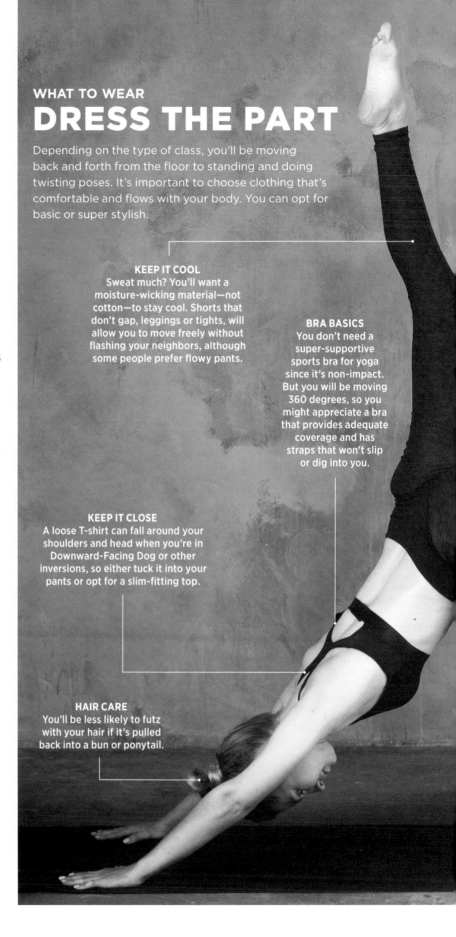

WHAT TO WEAR
DRESS THE PART

Depending on the type of class, you'll be moving back and forth from the floor to standing and doing twisting poses. It's important to choose clothing that's comfortable and flows with your body. You can opt for basic or super stylish.

KEEP IT COOL
Sweat much? You'll want a moisture-wicking material—not cotton—to stay cool. Shorts that don't gap, leggings or tights, will allow you to move freely without flashing your neighbors, although some people prefer flowy pants.

BRA BASICS
You don't need a super-supportive sports bra for yoga since it's non-impact. But you will be moving 360 degrees, so you might appreciate a bra that provides adequate coverage and has straps that won't slip or dig into you.

KEEP IT CLOSE
A loose T-shirt can fall around your shoulders and head when you're in Downward-Facing Dog or other inversions, so either tuck it into your pants or opt for a slim-fitting top.

HAIR CARE
You'll be less likely to futz with your hair if it's pulled back into a bun or ponytail.

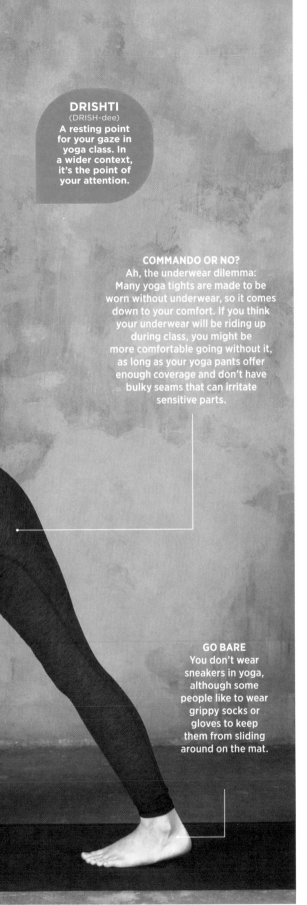

DRISHTI
(DRISH-dee)
A resting point for your gaze in yoga class. In a wider context, it's the point of your attention.

COMMANDO OR NO?
Ah, the underwear dilemma: Many yoga tights are made to be worn without underwear, so it comes down to your comfort. If you think your underwear will be riding up during class, you might be more comfortable going without it, as long as your yoga pants offer enough coverage and don't have bulky seams that can irritate sensitive parts.

GO BARE
You don't wear sneakers in yoga, although some people like to wear grippy socks or gloves to keep them from sliding around on the mat.

your awareness into your body. Next, depending on the style of yoga you're doing, you might do Sun Salutation (see pages 52-53) to warm up. In a flowing Vinyasa-style class, the speed will pick up and you'll add in other poses. As the class progresses, the flow may slow and you'll hold poses for several breaths. Next, you might do some balancing postures then move to the floor.

In more advanced classes, it's toward the end that you'll do inversions, such as head or shoulder stands (you never have to do any pose that you don't feel comfortable with). Many classes will build to a "peak" pose, which the postures you've done throughout the session have prepared you for. You'll end with some gentle poses followed by Savasana (resting pose) and possibly a meditation or some breathwork.

THERE'S NO EGO IN YOGA.

THE RIGHT ATTITUDE

So you've made it to class, you're surrounded by blocks, bolsters and blankets, and you're ready to get posing. You look around, noticing the cute outfit on the person in front of you or the hot guy in the corner. Maybe your competitive side starts to emerge. Newbie, meet your ego.

"I tell my beginners— and I mean this with loving kindness— 'Nobody cares what you can or can't do in yoga class. No one is watching you and thinking you're awesome or remarkably bad,'" says instructor Jason Crandell. "Being competitive doesn't serve a goal within your practice. There's no reward that comes from doing more or less than someone else."

While it's normal to feel competitive or insecure about your ability, you're in class to learn, says Crandell, so you have to let that stuff go and open yourself up to the experience. Be patient and have faith that you're right where you're supposed to be.

STEADY AS YOU FLOW

PICK YOUR POSE

You'll do a variety of moves in a typical yoga class—and they'll evolve as your skills improve, so you're always challenging yourself. Here, some yoga pose categories that you can expect to see just about every time and why they go way beyond stretching.

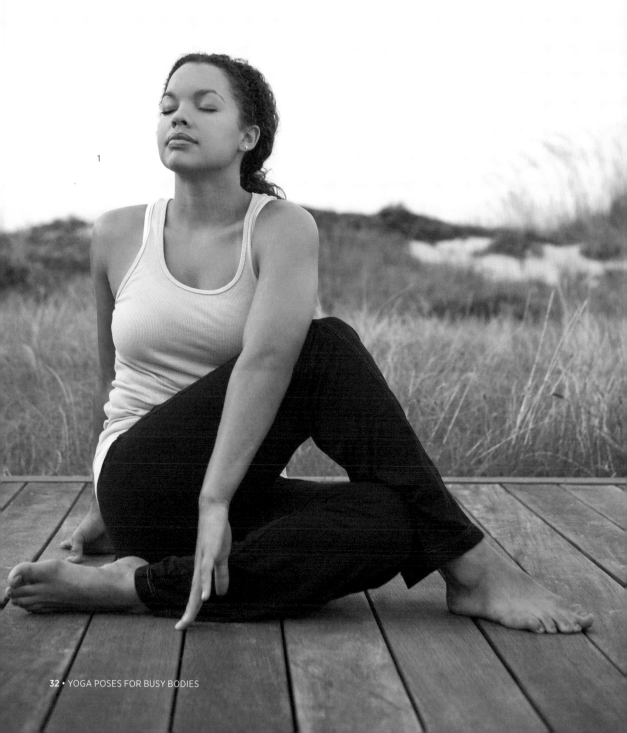

1

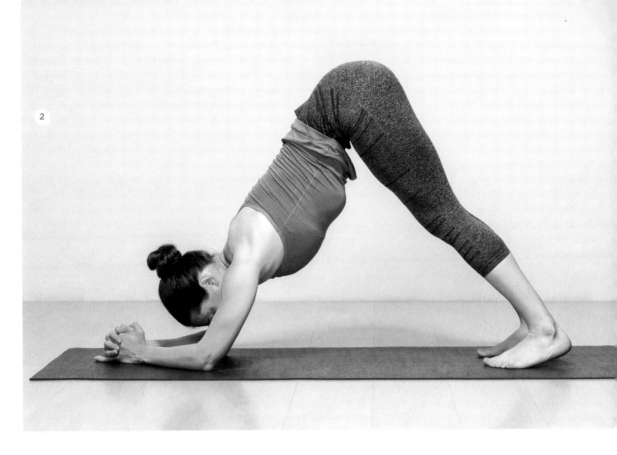

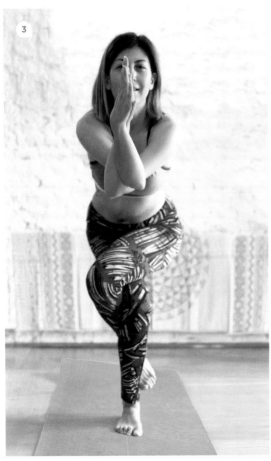

1 TWISTS Whether reclining on the floor, seated or standing, twisting moves, such as Half Lord of the Fishes Pose (photo 1), are excellent for the digestion because they're like an abdominal massage. They also help improve spine mobility, especially in the mid and upper back, and stretch those abdominal, low back and hip muscles that get tight. When you're twisting, visualize moving around a tall straight spindle, getting as much space as you can through your spine (elongating).

2 INVERSIONS Any move that takes the head below the heart is considered an inversion in yoga, whether that's a headstand or handstand, Downward-Facing Dog, Dolphin Pose (photo 2) or Child's Pose. Thanks to the increased blood (and oxygen) flow to the head, these poses are believed to be invigorating.

3 BINDS These tricky poses, such as Eagle (photo 3), are often combined with twists, balancing and other types of moves, which makes them complex. "The primary intention of binds is mobilizing the shoulder joint," says San Francisco yoga instructor Jason Crandell. "But secondarily, binds are about establishing and maintaining focus."

Q Do I have to do all the poses in class?

A If you're struggling with a particular posture, a good instructor will offer different options and show you how to modify or use blocks, says Adelle Daniels, owner of Yoga Mat Amarillo in Texas. "If it's just not accessible to you or you're tired, you can always choose Child's Pose or another posture that allows you to come back and connect with the breath," she says. "When you're ready, just jump back in."

Be warned: You may find certain poses a breeze on one day and difficult the next. Part of yoga is being able to accept where you are on that day, at that moment, and move on.

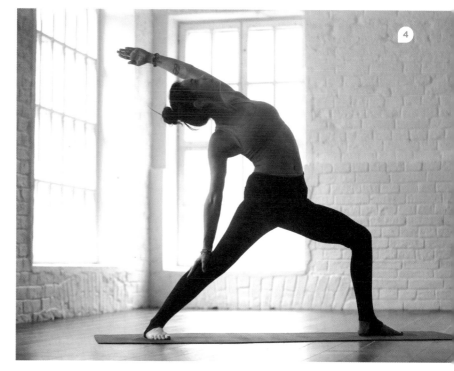

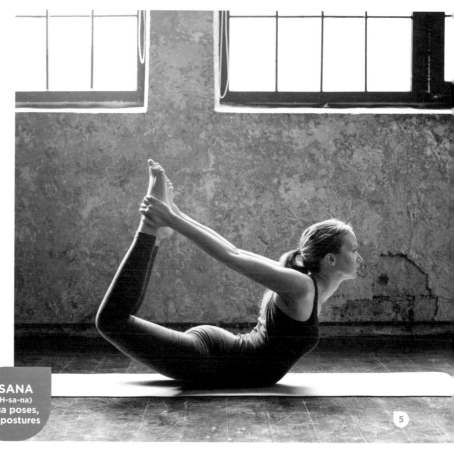

ASANA
(AH-sa-na)
Yoga poses,
aka postures

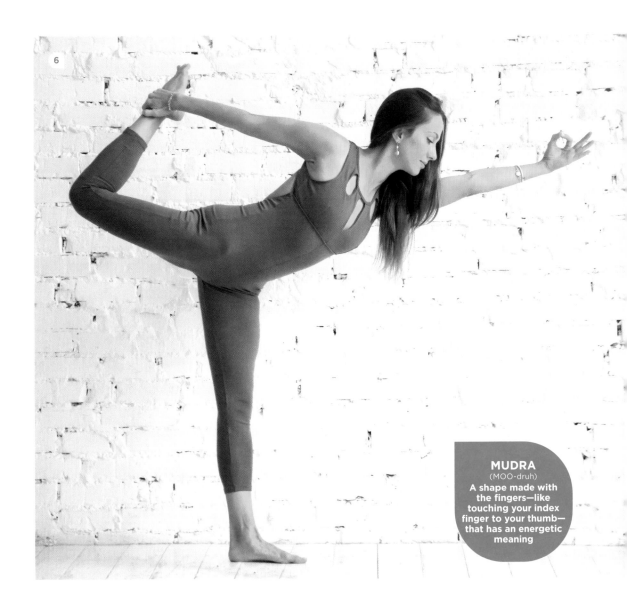

6

MUDRA
(MOO-druh)
**A shape made with
the fingers—like
touching your index
finger to your thumb—
that has an energetic
meaning**

4 SIDE BENDS These poses, such as Reverse Warrior (photo 4), help open up and stretch the sides of the rib cage. When the muscles in this area are tight, breathing can become restricted. People who sit crouched at a desk all day may find side bends really uncomfortable, but that's just a sign to keep doing them.

5 BACKBENDS Since so many people sit with their hips flexed and arms in front of them all day—or do exercises that primarily involve moving forward and back (walking, running, biking, the elliptical machine)—the muscles along the front of the body can get very shortened and tight. Backbends—even

something as simple as standing tall and leaning back slightly—help stretch the front of the body. These moves, such as Bow Pose (photo 5), are also often called chest or heart openers, since they release the chest and make it vulnerable.

6 BALANCE POSES Standing on one foot is an excellent opportunity to build hip strength and enhance those stabilizing muscles in your lower leg and ankle. Balance poses, such as King Dancer Pose (photo 6), are also an ideal way to challenge your mental focus. If your mind wanders, you'll have a harder time maintaining your balance.

GEAR
TOOL TIME

You don't need any equipment to do yoga, but sometimes the right accessories makes it easier to explore poses. Consider adding these objects to your practice.

MAT The most basic yoga accessory, these range from ⅛-inch to ¼-inch in thickness. Thin ones are more likely to slide around as you move, but going too thick will make it harder to balance, so look for one that's just right for you. Mats are usually 68 inches long, but tall yogis can find versions that go up to 85 inches.

BOLSTER These tube-shaped cushions are designed to support your body, but they can also provide an added balance challenge in certain poses. A rolled-up blanket can substitute as a bolster if necessary.

YOGA STRAP Can't quite touch your toes? That's where your strap comes in. It bridges the gap between where you are and where you want to be.

BLOCK Yes, it will help you get into poses that your flexibility might not normally allow you to access, but it also does double duty as a self-massage tool.

YOGA WHEEL The wheel has been reinvented over and over again—and now it's for yoga. These help you stretch out tight areas, but they're also good for getting into backbends.

YOGA TOWEL Sweat much? Top your mat with a soft towel. Look for one that's specially designed to go on top of a mat so it won't slip as you move.

SANDBAGS Weighted blankets are all the rage for calming, and some studios offer sandbags that you can drape over your hips or chest while you're resting in Savasana or during a restorative or Yoga Nidra class.

GRIP SOCKS Nonslip yoga socks help you stick to your mat and can give beginners more confidence.

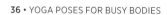

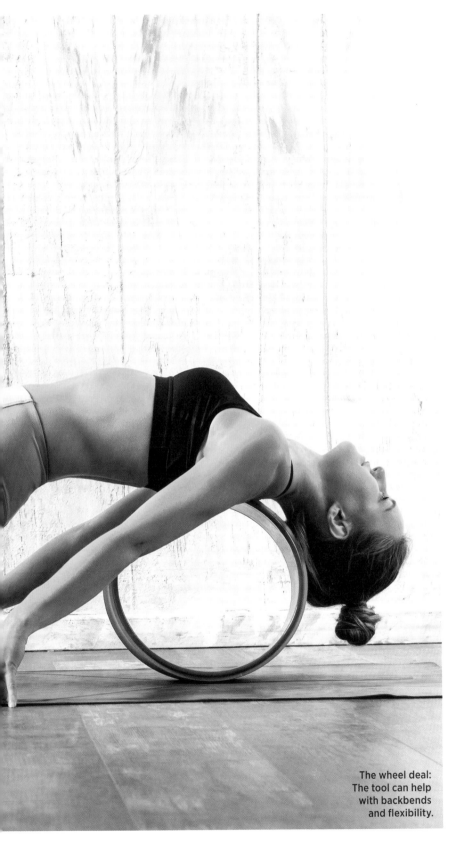

The wheel deal:
The tool can help
with backbends
and flexibility.

Q What's up
with the chanting?

A "There are so many
different traditions
and philosophies of
yoga and, depending
on the class or teacher,
you may experience
different ways that
chanting is used," says
Yoga Mat Amarillo's
Adelle Daniels. Some
people repeat the
Sanskrit word "*om*,"
while others may
chant a phrase. "I use
chanting occasionally
at the beginning or
end of class and it's
really just another way
to bring awareness to
the moment and to
help calm and center
everyone." If you
prefer to sit silently,
though, the yoga
police aren't going
to come and kick
you out.

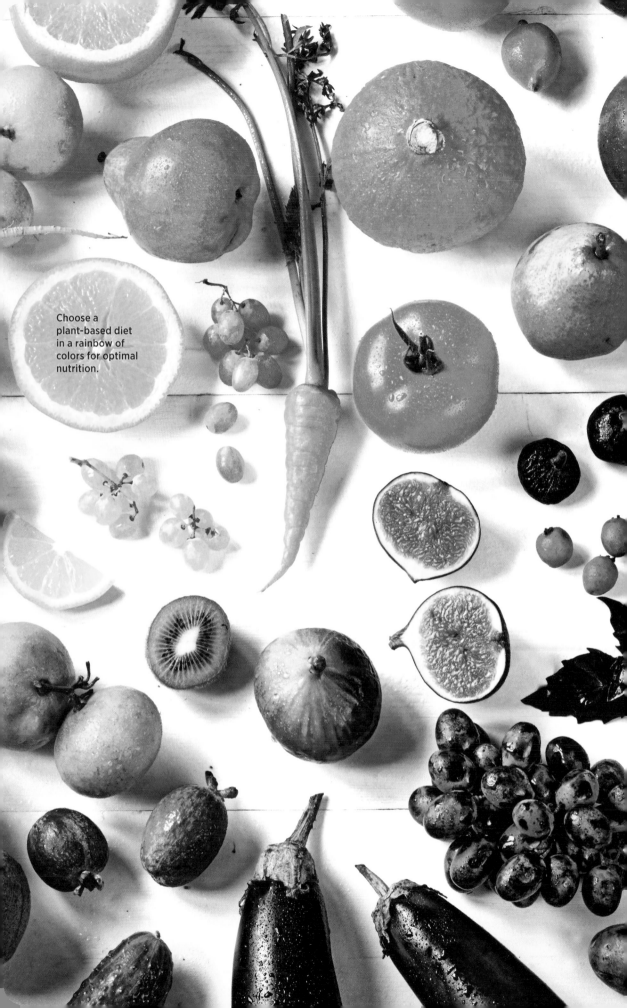

Choose a
plant-based diet
in a rainbow of
colors for optimal
nutrition.

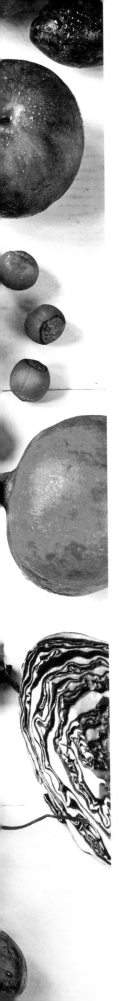

EAT LIKE A YOGI

TAKE YOUR YOGA PRACTICE OFF THE MAT AND INTO THE KITCHEN TO SEE HOW IT CAN CHANGE YOUR RELATIONSHIP WITH FOOD.

One of the wonderful things about yoga is the positive ripple effect it can have on every other aspect of your life, including your diet. "Any practice that brings consciousness to the body can start to trickle down to your lifestyle," says holistic nutrition coach and Ayurvedic counselor Noelle Renée Kovary, author of *The Self-Healing Revolution: Modern-Day Ayurveda With Recipes and Tools for Intuitive Living.* "Breathing deeply into your belly, the way you do in yoga, helps you quiet everything else so all you feel is your body. If you take this breathwork and consciousness off the mat, it can help you choose better foods as well."

While there is no "yoga diet," there are some eating practices and behaviors that are popular in the yoga community (we're not talking about juicing or other fads). These are ways of eating that can actually improve your health and help you become more aware of habits that may no longer be serving you. Check out the following, see what works best for you and your lifestyle—and remember to always use your body's innate wisdom as your guide.

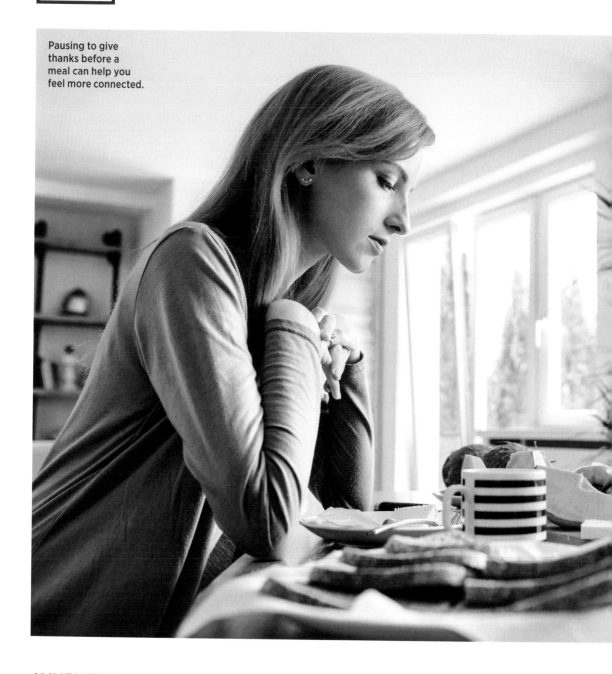

Pausing to give thanks before a meal can help you feel more connected.

AYURVEDA

This system of healing comes from the Vedas, ancient texts that serve as the foundation of yoga. Ayurveda is the oldest health-care system practice that's still used today, says Boston–based Kara Lydon, RD, author of the self-published e-book *Nourish Your Namaste: How Nutrition and Yoga Can Support Digestion, Immunity, Energy and Relaxation.* Although each person's specific "ideal" diet varies based on their dosha, in general, Ayurvedic nutrition involves eating based on the

seasons and choosing mostly plant-based foods. "In the winter, you should focus on root vegetables, warm foods and hearty comfort foods like sweet potatoes, carrots, parsnips, butternut squash, beets, turnips and kohlrabi," explains Lydon. "In the hot summer months, you should focus on cooling foods like salads, fresh fruits and vegetables, yogurt, cilantro and coconut." Some practitioners also recommend getting the six Ayurvedic tastes at each meal—sweet, sour, salty, bitter, astringent and pungent. (For more on Ayurveda, see page 20.)

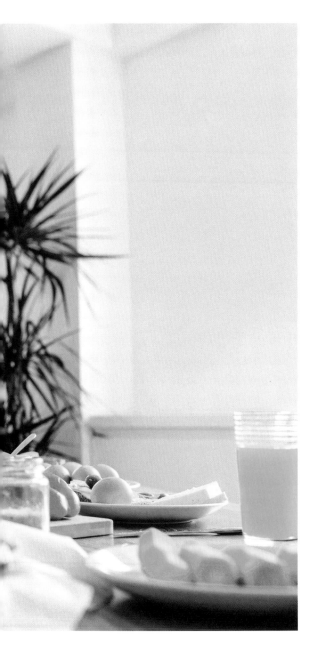

Eating a primarily plant-based diet does have health benefits, though. According to the *American Journal of Clinical Nutrition*, vegans tend to get more healthy fat, fiber and other nutrients, but can fall short when it comes to calcium. Still, you have to decide what works best for you.

MINDFUL EATING

For years, dietitians and nutritionists have advised eating mindfully, which just means slowing down, listening to what your body is telling you, and using all of your senses to enjoy your food. According to a review published in the journal *Current Obesity Reports*, mindful eating may help you grow more in tune with hunger and satiety, decrease cravings and reward-driven eating, and help you realize when external triggers are prompting hunger. "Yoga teaches you how to honor your hunger and fullness cues, knowing when and how much to eat and what foods might feel best in your body," Lydon says.

GRATITUDE FOR MEALS

Many different religions encourage saying some form of prayer before eating, and yoga is similar in that regard. "It can help you cultivate a relationship to a higher universal power that makes you feel more connected and grateful, and that practice can extend to eating," Lydon explains. And it doesn't have to be a traditional, "God"-focused prayer. You might pause to think about where the food came from and who grew and harvested it or visualize how the food is going to nourish you. It's really an opportunity to practice mindful eating.

"CLEAN" EATING

As you become more aware of your body through yoga, you may also notice how it reacts to certain foods. Some may make you feel energized and strong, others may leave you feeling sluggish or bloated. This awareness may prompt you to eliminate or limit certain foods, including gluten, soy, dairy or other options. Although this isn't inherently a bad thing, it can become a slippery slope and even lead to disordered eating. If your choices start to negatively impact your life and relationships, you know something's not working. See a registered dietitian or therapist who specializes in eating disorders for help.

VEGANISM

"There's a common belief that in order to be a 'good yogi,' you have to be a vegan or vegetarian," Lydon says. This is based on the concept of *ahimsa*, which means non-violence or non-harming. But Lydon believes shunning animal products is a misinterpretation. "Non-harming also means non-harming of the self. If you gave up meat and realized that you were losing weight, felt weaker and tired, and had low energy, then you would be doing harm to yourself by adopting a vegetarian lifestyle."

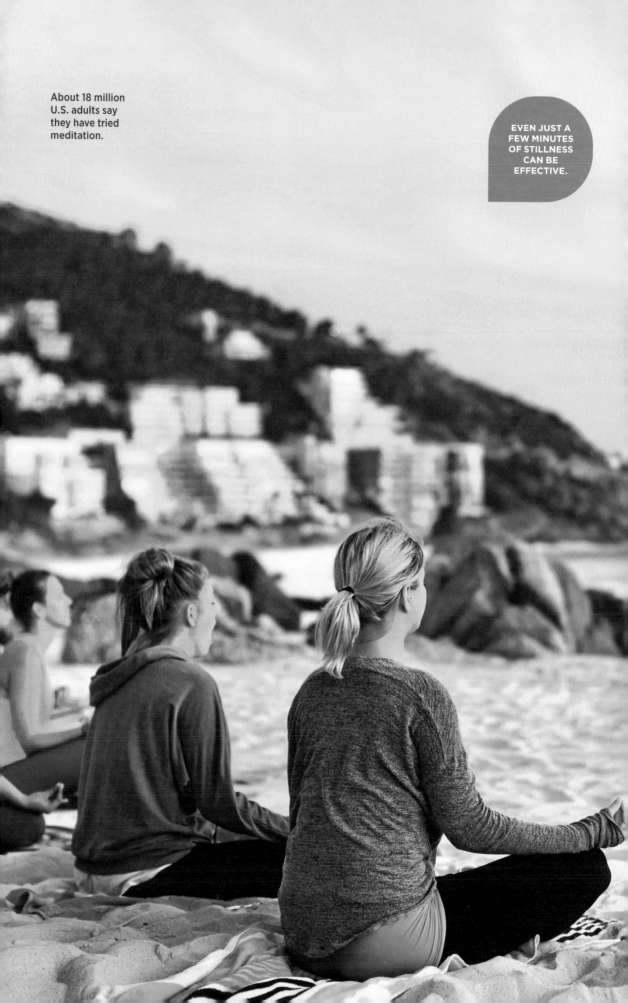

About 18 million U.S. adults say they have tried meditation.

EVEN JUST A FEW MINUTES OF STILLNESS CAN BE EFFECTIVE.

PEACE OUT

YOGA TEACHES US HOW TO BE MINDFUL IN STILLNESS AND MOVEMENT. HERE'S HOW TO USE MEDITATION TO GET MORE OUT OF YOUR POSES—AND LIFE.

Meditation and yoga are so intertwined that many people have a hard time distinguishing them: You can't think of one without the other coming to mind. And while you can meditate or do yoga separately, they go hand-in-hand for good reason. "Meditation is one of the eight limbs of yoga practice," explains Jessica Matthews, DBH, professor of integrative wellness at Point Loma Nazarene University in San Diego.

"Asana practice was started as a way to prepare and be able to sit for meditation," adds Amy Ippoliti, E-RYT, a yoga instructor based in Boulder, Colorado. "Your body is nice and warm and your hips are open, so you're able to sit comfortably. In turn, meditation allows your yoga practice to be a bit more focused and less distracted, too."

Even more powerful is how the two can both benefit other areas of your life. "Both yoga and meditation allow for the cultivation of enhanced awareness physically, mentally, emotionally and spiritually," Matthews says. That consciousness helps reduce stress, improve focus and boost productivity, while reducing reactivity. It allows you to better stay above the fray of life, whether it's negative thoughts and emotions or getting caught up in the frenzy of daily "to-do's."

THE PERKS OF PRESENCE

Yoga has numerous and diverse health benefits—thanks to the physical movement and mindfulness aspects. And meditation, even with its inherent stillness, continues to rack up impressive research, proving its worth in the following ways.

1 A SHARPER MIND Studies suggest that meditation changes brain regions involved in self-control and executive function. This means it may help reduce knee-jerk reactions, increase the chances you'll reach your goals, boost mood and promote focus. "We are all overstimulated and plugged in and completely at the whim of social media and information feeds. There is no pause button—ever," Ippoliti says. "Meditation allows us to have that pause."

Other studies show meditation may help with working memory, which is a short-term cache for things like recalling the name of a colleague's partner or remembering to pick up more paper towels when you stop at the supermarket. Meditation may even help offset neurodegenerative diseases by increasing the volume of gray matter in the brain, but more research is necessary.

2 LOWER BLOOD PRESSURE Meditation appears to reduce systolic blood pressure (the top number). Researchers believe it may dim the body's reaction to stress, in turn lowering heart rate and blood pressure.

3 IMPROVED MENTAL HEALTH Various studies find a link between meditation and reduced stress, anxiety and depression. "When you use things like the breath to anchor yourself in the present moment, you induce the relaxation response," Matthews explains. "I can't think of anyone who wouldn't benefit from this." Meditation also allows you to find that space between your thoughts and the feelings and emotions you attach to them.

4 SLOWER AGING A combination of meditation, yoga and pranayama (breathwork) may prevent chronic diseases and slow aging, according to a 2017 study published in the journal *Oxidative Medicine and Cellular Longevity*. Researchers found that practicing the three for a total of 90 minutes

five days a week improved biomarkers of cellular aging. "Making yoga and meditation an integral part of our lifestyle may hold the key to delay aging or to age gracefully, prevent onset of multifactorial complex lifestyle diseases, promote mental, physical and reproductive health and prolong a youthful, healthy life," the study authors concluded.

5 GREATER CREATIVITY AND PATIENCE Many people report that meditation helps them "unplug" from their fast-paced lives. "That ability to slow down helps declutter the mind," Ippoliti says. "When I meditate I feel I'm more creative, I get ideas more easily, and I'm calmer, more patient and less likely to direct anger at others."

PUT YOUR MIND TO IT

"Meditation can take various forms, and it's so powerful no matter how you practice it. Plus, it's always accessible," Matthews says. "It's not about clearing your mind, but being anchored in the present moment." Various meditation approaches utilize different elements of repetition as a way to anchor the mind.

BREATHING MEDITATION Matthews recommends a breath-based meditation for beginners, since it tends to be the most accessible approach. Simply sit with your eyes closed or gently open (although having them closed often makes it easier to focus). Then start to observe your breath, without judgment or trying to change it. If your mind wanders, gently bring your attention back to your breath. Try this meditation from Matthews: Begin by noticing your breath moving in and out of your body. Once you feel settled, start counting your breaths: inhale 1, exhale 2, inhale 3, exhale 4. Then start over at 1, continuing until your time is up.

MANTRA MEDITATION A mantra is a statement or affirmation that you repeat. "Not only is that bringing your attention to one thing rather than ruminating or going off on 'thinking journeys,' there is a quality to the mantra—it means something," Ippoliti says. Those words can help you cultivate a way that you want to behave, or a mindset you wish to hold. Traditionally mantras are in Sanskrit, but they don't have to be. Just choose a word or phrase such as "I am enough," "I am strong" or "Less is more" (or coin your own)—then sit and repeat it silently to yourself.

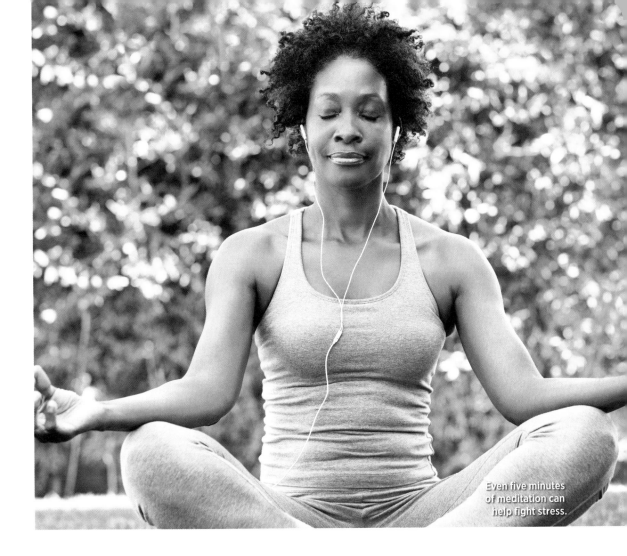

Even five minutes of meditation can help fight stress.

SENSORY MEDITATION Incorporate one or more of your senses into your practice. Notice the ambient sounds, how your body feels, the scents in the air, any flavors in your mouth, and even picture the space around you with your eyes closed.

LOVING-KINDNESS MEDITATION This specific style of meditation helps foster compassion toward others and yourself. You can find a script or guided audio online. In general, the practice starts by receiving loving-kindness for yourself, then sending it to loved ones, people you've had difficult interactions with and others.

VISUALIZATION Although not technically meditation, "visualization cultivates present awareness," says Matthews, who considers it among stress-management strategies and mindfulness practices. Try picturing a serene scene, such as a mountaintop or beach, to promote relaxation.

MAXIMIZE YOUR MEDITATION TIME

"It isn't so important that the conditions be perfect for you to start a practice, but that you start," Ippoliti says. Don't worry about having a meditation cushion or being able to sit in lotus pose or carving out 20 minutes. Start with one minute—yep, just 60 seconds—and go from there. The duration doesn't matter, although increasing it over time will boost the benefits, she adds.

What Ippoliti does recommend is consistency. "Think of it as filling your spiritual bank account," she says. "Every time you practice, you are making a deposit. If you only meditate three times in your life, that won't accrue much interest. But if you log a lot of hours, then during the times when you can't practice, that bank account will be there for you to tap into." If you can't do an "official" quiet meditation, try to at least create space for mindfulness in your daily routine. Practice it as your coffee is brewing, while you do the dishes or any time you can take a pause.

45

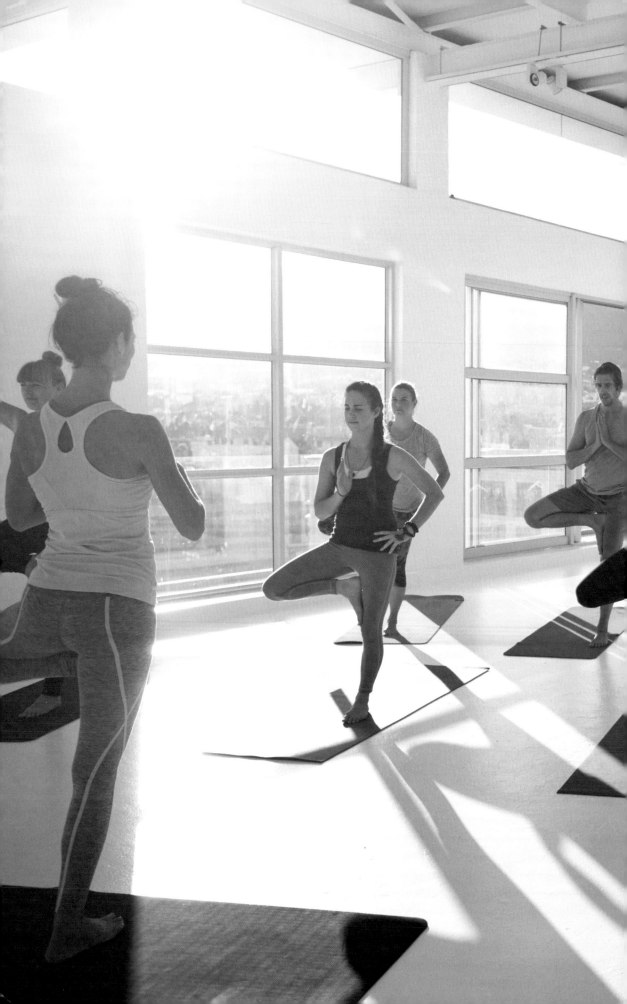

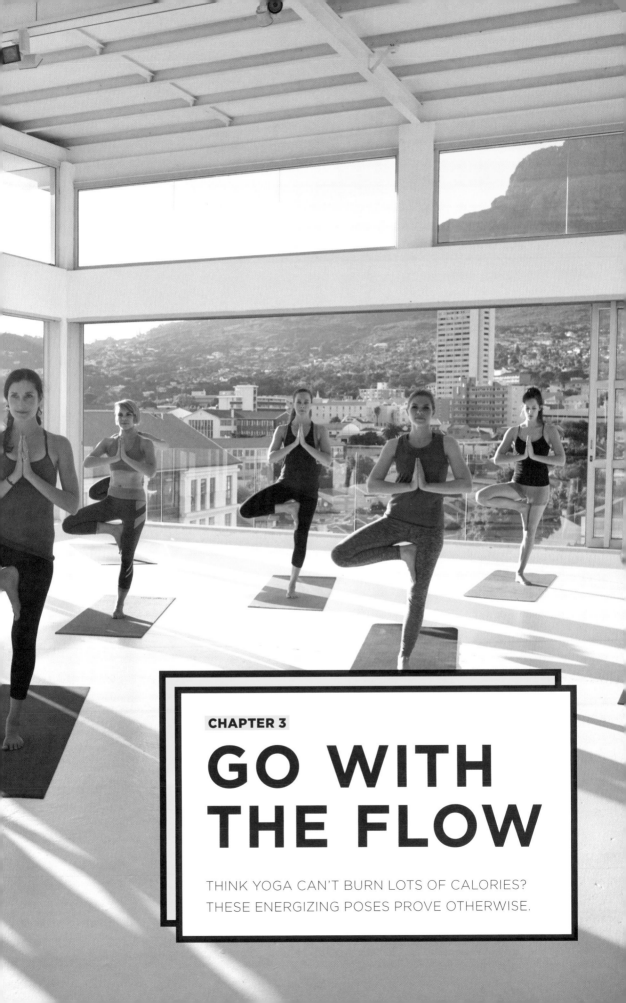

CHAPTER 3

GO WITH THE FLOW

THINK YOGA CAN'T BURN LOTS OF CALORIES?
THESE ENERGIZING POSES PROVE OTHERWISE.

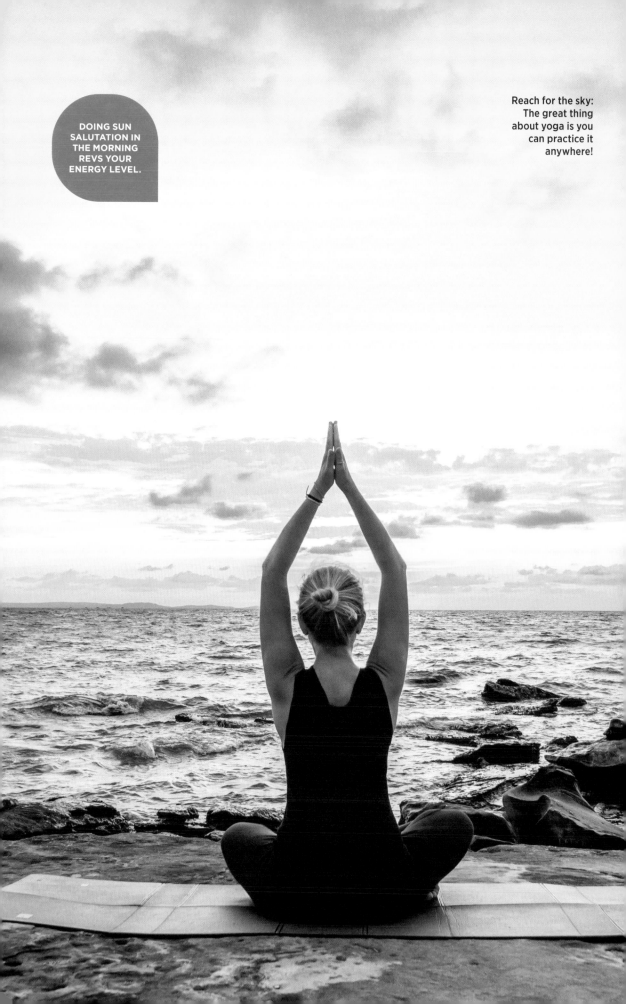

DOING SUN SALUTATION IN THE MORNING REVS YOUR ENERGY LEVEL.

Reach for the sky: The great thing about yoga is you can practice it anywhere!

HERE COMES THE SUN

THIS TRADITIONAL SERIES OF FLOWING MOVES SERVES AS A WAY TO WARM UP THE ENTIRE BODY AS WELL AS A CHANCE TO HONOR THE NATURAL WORLD.

Like so many other ancient practices, yoga holds special reverence for nature, animals and the elements (space, air, fire, water and earth) because people back then lived more in rhythm with nature. Many yoga poses are named after animals or celestial bodies. And one flowing series found in many yoga practices is perhaps the most famous of all. Surya Namaskar—aka Sun Salutation—means "bowing to the sun." It serves as a warm-up for the poses to come; as you go through the moves you'll notice that it works virtually every muscle and joint in your body. But you can also use it as a moving practice of gratitude for another sunrise, another day, another chance to live harmoniously— or just to rev up your heart rate. In some traditions, you're supposed to do 108 rounds of Sun Salutation when seasons change or to mark a new year (108 is a sacred number in the Hindu religion).

There are different variations of Sun Salutation but the one on these pages is the most basic (aka

Surya Namaskar A). In it you start standing, move to the floor and end up standing again. "You're really warming up the spine, doing forward folds and backbends," says yoga instructor Allison Candelaria, E-RYT, owner of Soul Yoga in Oklahoma City. "By inhaling or exhaling with each movement, you're connecting the mind, body and breath, which brings blood, oxygen and energy to all your cells."

The Sun Salutation series engages the entire body.

LEARN THE BASICS.

ON CUE

The following tips on form will help you get more out of every yoga pose.

1 GROUND YOURSELF When standing, distribute your weight between the big and little toes and heel so you're not rolling in or out on your foot. Lift the inner arch of your feet off the floor. If your hands are on the floor, press your palms and knuckles into the mat. Think of "gripping" the mat without moving your hands.

2 STAY LONG Unless the pose requires something different, try to keep your spine elongated, from the tip of your head to tailbone.

3 PULL YOUR RIBS DOWN Think of drawing the bottom of the rib cage and top of hip bones together. This engages the abs, enables better breathing and creates stability through the torso. It also keeps you from overextending the spine.

4 FIND A FOCAL POINT Maintain your focus on your breath and body. In balancing poses, you'll need to find a specific point on the floor or wall (something that's not moving) to help you keep from wobbling. This is called a *drishti* in Sanskrit.

5 GET COMFORTABLE WITH OPPOSITION In most poses, many things happen at once. You may be extending your limbs in opposite directions and rooting into the mat while rising up. This is part of yoga's dynamic energy.

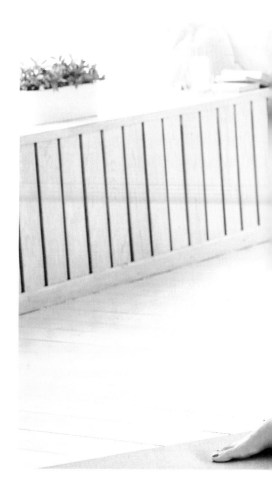

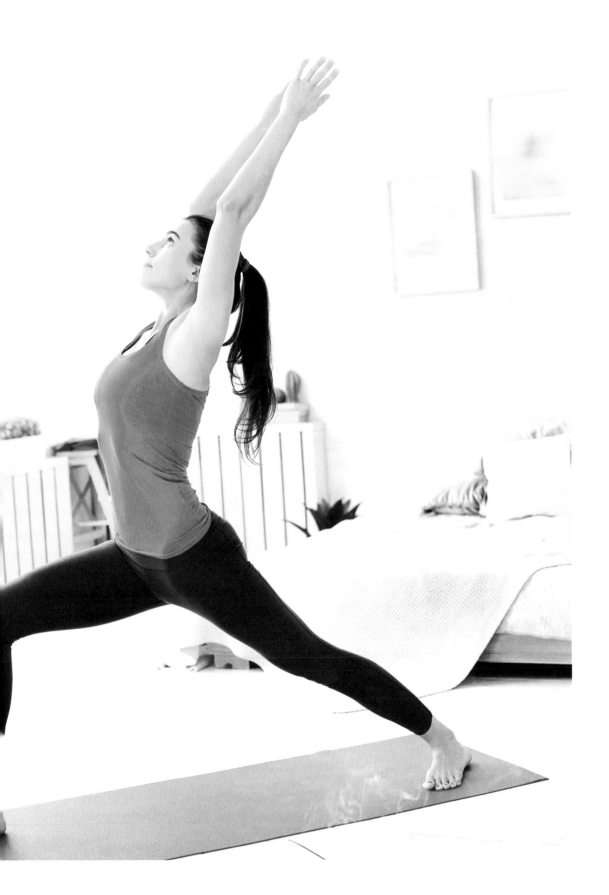

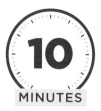

10 MINUTES

HOW TO DO IT
SUN SALUTATION

Do several rounds of the following as its own flow or as a warm-up to some of the other routines in this book. If you have to stop and rest at some point, just hold the posture or rest in Downward-Facing Dog (below right) or Child's Pose (see page 117), then continue when you're ready. Aim to move mindfully without rushing it. As you get familiar with the poses, you'll be able to pick up the pace.

MOUNTAIN POSE (TADASANA)
Stand with your feet together or slightly apart, palms pressed together in front of your chest. Notice the sensation of your feet grounding to the mat, your weight evenly balanced between your big and little toes and your heels. Focus your attention on your body and breath, inhaling and exhaling through the nose for several breaths before you begin **(1)**. Inhale as you raise your arms overhead.

STANDING FORWARD BEND (UTTANASANA)
Exhale as you dive forward from the hips, keeping your back flat until you have to round at the bottom, neck relaxed **(2)**. You can keep your knees slightly bent throughout the move to protect your back, or if you don't have the hamstring flexibility to keep the knees straight.

STANDING HALF FORWARD BEND (ARDHA UTTANASANA)
Inhale as you look forward, rising up slightly and flattening your back. Let your fingertips graze the mat or your shins **(not shown)**. Think of a light that's attached to your sternum shining forward. Exhale as you fold over your legs again.

LOW LUNGE (ANJANEYASANA)
Inhale as you step your right foot back into a deep lunge. The front knee should be aligned over your front ankle. Lift your chest and look forward, keeping hands on floor **(3)**.

PLANK POSE (PHALAKASANA)
With palms shoulder-width apart on the mat, exhale as you step your left leg back to meet your right. Your body should be in a straight line from head to heels, shoulders over palms **(4)**. If this is too challenging, lower your knees to the floor. Press away from the mat and inhale again.

FOUR-LIMBED STAFF POSE (CHATURANGA DANDASANA)
Exhale as you shift yourself forward on your toes and lift your sternum. Bend your elbows no more than 90 degrees, keeping them tucked to your sides **(5)**. If you're a beginner, start with your knees on the mat. Slowly lower yourself all the way to the mat.

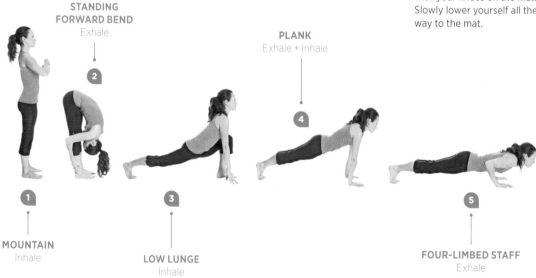

STANDING FORWARD BEND
Exhale
2

PLANK
Exhale + Inhale
4

1
MOUNTAIN
Inhale

3
LOW LUNGE
Inhale

5
FOUR-LIMBED STAFF
Exhale

COBRA POSE (BHUJANGASANA)

Inhale as you lift your head and chest off the floor, drawing your shoulders away from your ears. You don't have to lift very far. Some people may be able to lift more of their torso and almost straighten the arms **(6)**, but it doesn't have to be a big lift. Usually by the third or fourth time through the series you'll be able to lift higher off the mat.

DOWNWARD-FACING DOG (ADHO MUKHA SVANASANA)

Exhale as you lift your hips and press your chest toward your legs, forming an inverted "V" **(7)**. (From Cobra you can also lower your chest to the floor and come to all fours, with wrists under shoulders and knees under hips. Then curl your toes under and lift your hips so you're in an inverted V position.) It's OK if your heels don't touch the mat or your knees are bent. Press your chest toward your feet and let your neck relax. Think about rotating your arms outward (turn your inner elbows forward) as your shoulder blades draw down your back, and press your hands into the mat. Take a few breaths or keep moving.

LOW LUNGE (ANJANEYASANA)

On an inhale, step your right foot forward into a deep lunge, with the knee aligned over the ankle. Lift your chest and look forward **(8)**.

STANDING FORWARD BEND (UTTANASANA)

Exhale as you step your feet together (or place them hip-width apart) and fold over your legs, letting your spine round and your neck relax **(9)**.

MOUNTAIN POSE (TADASANA)

Inhale as you slowly rise up and sweep your arms overhead; look up at your hands. Then exhale as you bring your palms together in front of your heart **(10)**. Repeat sequence on opposite side.

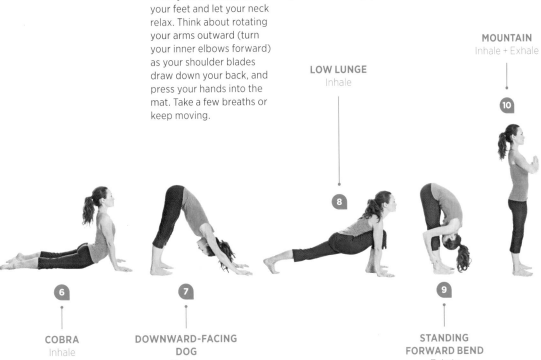

MOUNTAIN
Inhale + Exhale

LOW LUNGE
Inhale

10

8

6

9

COBRA
Inhale

DOWNWARD-FACING DOG
Exhale

STANDING FORWARD BEND
Exhale

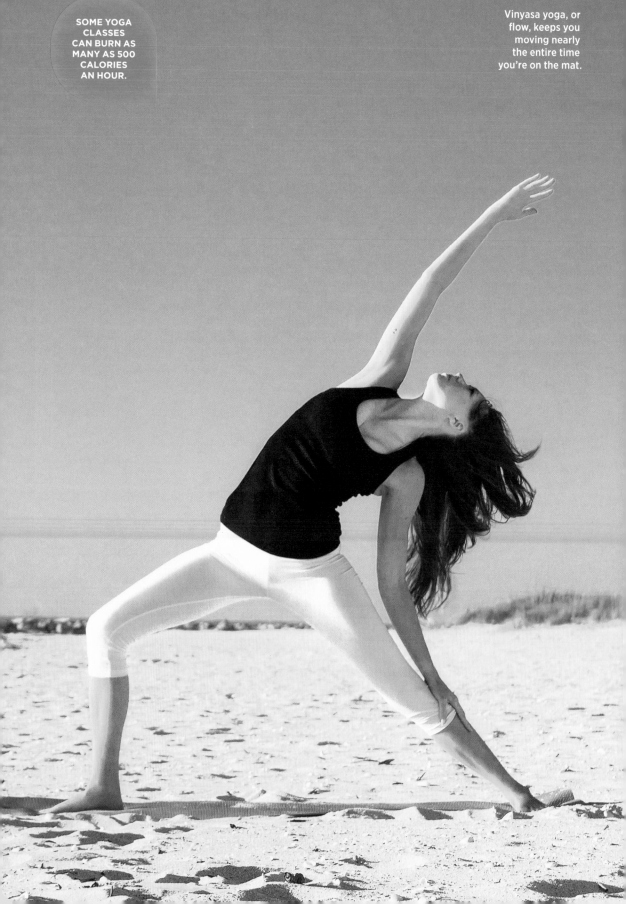

SOME YOGA CLASSES CAN BURN AS MANY AS 500 CALORIES AN HOUR.

Vinyasa yoga, or flow, keeps you moving nearly the entire time you're on the mat.

ENERGIZE YOUR YOGA ROUTINE

THIS FLOWING, INTERVAL-STYLE WORKOUT TAKES A PAGE FROM REGULAR FITNESS CLASSES. USE IT TO FEEL MORE AWAKE AND BURN EXTRA CALORIES.

If you're into fitness you're probably familiar with the term HIIT, which stands for high-intensity interval training. It intersperses higher-intensity bursts of exercise (think: sprints or hills) with slower-paced recovery periods. It's all the rage since it provides serious results (fat loss, cardiovascular benefits) in less time—as little as 10 minutes. And while yoga is usually known for its laid-back pace, many people don't have time to do yoga *and* cardio *and* lift weights, so they want to feel like they got a "workout" doing yoga. As a result, faster-paced classes—yoga HIIT or yoga intervals—are gaining popularity. "Yoga HIIT is appealing because you get more bang for your buck," says yoga instructor and personal trainer Kirsten Beverley-Waters, RYT, who teaches a yoga HIIT fusion class in West Falmouth, Maine.

While you might feel like you're burning a ton of calories in some yoga classes, a research review found yoga burns about the same amount as walking at a moderate 3 mph pace on a flat surface. That's about 230 calories an hour (for a 145-pound woman). Doing a faster-paced flow, such as Sun Salutation (see pages 52-53), will double that calorie burn, on average. Now we're talking!

"Sometimes those slow-flow classes can get stagnant," says yoga instructor and teacher-trainer Allison Candelaria, E-RYT, owner of Soul Yoga in Oklahoma City. "By increasing blood flow and engaging the muscles in a new way, interval yoga can be a great supplement to regular Hatha classes and provide a new challenge."

USE THIS TRICK TO WAKE UP!

BREATHE FIRE

Many yogis do pranayama, or breathwork, every morning as part of a ritual to help them start their day. Ujjayi breathing (see page 29) is one type of pranayama that can boost energy. But if you're really trying to wake up, try kapalabhati ("breath of fire" or "skull shining breath").

"While it's energizing it's also very calming," says yoga instructor Allison Candelaria. "It might take you a few times to get used to it, though." (Do it on an empty stomach; if you're pregnant or have a heart condition or emphysema stick with ujjayi breathing.)

Try it: Sit tall, eyes closed. Start with ujjayi breathing. After several breaths, inhale, then quickly draw your belly in, forcing the air out through your nose. Let your belly relax on its own as you inhale naturally, then repeat. Do 10 breaths, then exhale any remaining air out of your lungs; inhale and hold for five counts. Do three rounds. (If you feel dizzy, stop and breathe normally.)

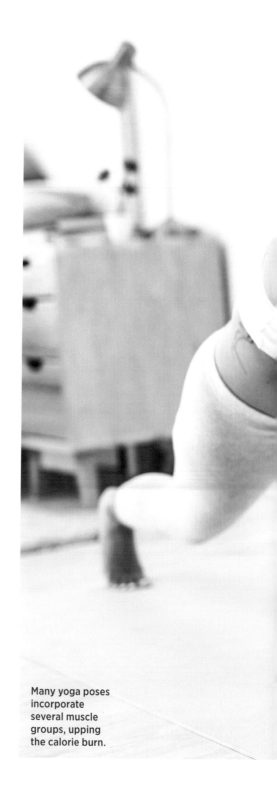

Many yoga poses incorporate several muscle groups, upping the calorie burn.

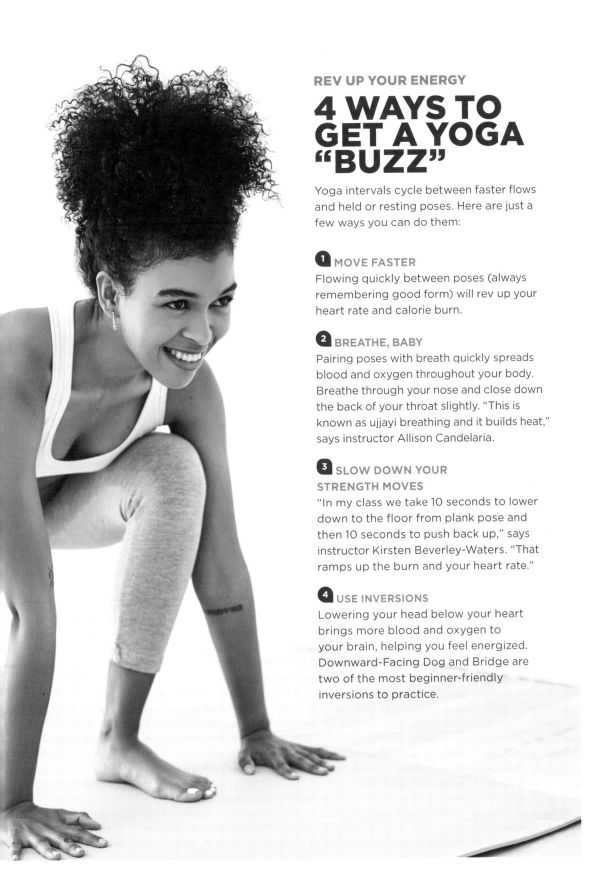

4 WAYS TO GET A YOGA "BUZZ"

Yoga intervals cycle between faster flows and held or resting poses. Here are just a few ways you can do them:

1 MOVE FASTER
Flowing quickly between poses (always remembering good form) will rev up your heart rate and calorie burn.

2 BREATHE, BABY
Pairing poses with breath quickly spreads blood and oxygen throughout your body. Breathe through your nose and close down the back of your throat slightly. "This is known as ujjayi breathing and it builds heat," says instructor Allison Candelaria.

3 SLOW DOWN YOUR STRENGTH MOVES
"In my class we take 10 seconds to lower down to the floor from plank pose and then 10 seconds to push back up," says instructor Kirsten Beverley-Waters. "That ramps up the burn and your heart rate."

4 USE INVERSIONS
Lowering your head below your heart brings more blood and oxygen to your brain, helping you feel energized. Downward-Facing Dog and Bridge are two of the most beginner-friendly inversions to practice.

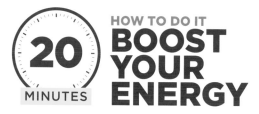

20 MINUTES

HOW TO DO IT
BOOST YOUR ENERGY

The following workout, created by instructor Allison Candelaria and demonstrated by Trisha Curling, RYT, owner of Ani O Yoga in Toronto, Canada, uses quick movement, rhythmic breathing paced with poses, and some inversions to boost energy. Warm up with three to five rounds of Sun Salutation (see pages 52-53) and for even more oomph, add a round (or more) between each of the intervals below. Go through the two intervals below in order and then repeat them once or twice as time allows.

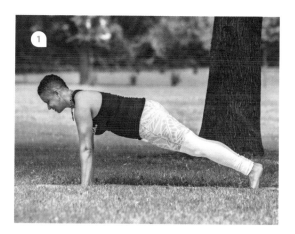

INTERVAL 1

PLANK TO DOWNWARD-FACING DOG

1 PLANK (PHALAKASANA)
Get on all fours, wrists under your shoulders and knees under hips. Lift knees and step one foot back at a time, so your body is straight from head to heels **(1)**. Hold for one full breath. (Keep your knees down to make this easier, if needed.)

2 DOWNWARD-FACING DOG (ADHO MUKHA SVANASANA)
From plank, lift your hips so your body forms an inverted V. Your legs should be straight or almost straight, heels reaching toward the ground (they may not make it). Press your chest toward your feet, think about rotating your inner elbows toward each other and draw your shoulder blades down. Engage your quadriceps muscles (this will lift your kneecaps). For more of a challenge, raise your right leg up into a Three-Legged Downward-Facing Dog **(2)**.

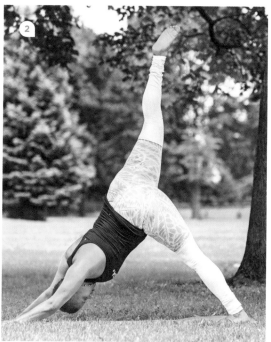

Hold for one full breath. Move back and forth between Plank and Downward-Facing Dog five times. Keep one leg raised the entire time or switch legs each time. As you get comfortable, inhale into Plank Pose and exhale into Downward-Facing Dog.

3 RECOVER: EXTENDED PUPPY POSE (UTTANA SHISHOSANA)
From Downward-Facing Dog, return to all fours and walk your hands forward, keeping your hips over your knees. Once your arms are extended, lower your forehead to the mat **(3)**. Hold this position for three to five breaths. Do a Sun Salutation, or move on to Interval 2.

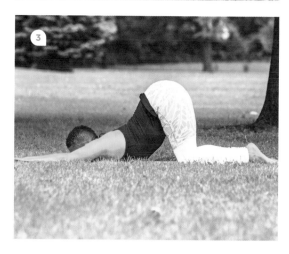

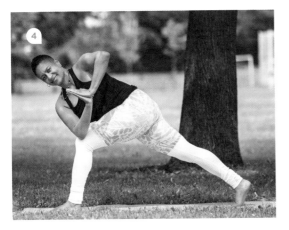

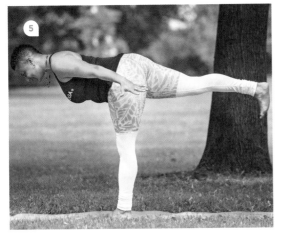

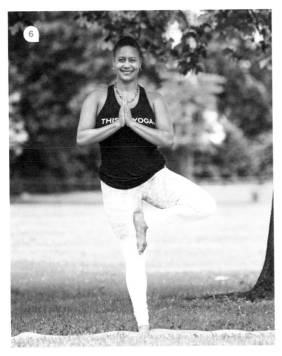

TWISTED CRESCENT TO AIRPLANE

4 TWISTED CRESCENT (PARIVRTTA ANJANEYASANA)

Stand with feet hip-width apart, then step right foot back and bend left knee 90 degrees so the thigh is parallel to the ground and the knee is aligned over ankle. (Feet remain parallel and hip-distance apart, even though you're in a lunge, for stability. If your feet look like you're walking a tightrope, move your back foot out from the center.) Place palms together in front of your chest; twist your upper body to the left and lean over, locking the right elbow outside the left knee if possible **(4)**. Try to keep your hands in the center of your chest; if you can't get your elbow outside your knee, don't force it. Hold here for one full breath.

5 AIRPLANE (DEKASANA)

Slowly turn back to the center and shift your weight to the left foot, pushing off your back foot. Bend over from your hips so your torso is parallel to the ground and extend your arms at your sides or bring them forward, palms facing each other. Lift the right leg behind you until it's parallel to the ground **(5)**, or rest your back foot lightly on the ground to help you stay balanced. Keep your hips squared to the mat (don't let the hip on the rear leg hike up). Hold here for one full breath.

Move back and forth between these poses five times, then switch sides and repeat. As you get comfortable, exhale for Twisted Crescent Pose and inhale as you move into Airplane.

6 RECOVER: TREE POSE (VRKSASANA)

Slowly rise up from Airplane and stand with feet hip-width apart. Shift weight to your right leg and place the bottom of your left foot against the inside of your calf or upper thigh (or leave your toes on the ground and rest your heel against your ankle; don't rest your foot against the inside of your knee, which can stress the ligaments). Place your palms together in front of your chest **(6)** or raise arms overhead. Hold for five breaths, keeping your hips even (don't sink into your standing leg) and pressing your foot and leg against each other to help you grow taller. Lower left leg to mat and repeat on opposite side.

Add in one (or more) rounds of Sun Salutation, or go back to Interval 1 and repeat from the beginning.

As you gain experience in yoga, you can start to play around with poses that you enjoy and that feel good linked together in a flowing series. In this way you can create your own interval-type flow and change it up each time, depending on how you feel or what your body needs. One of the joys of yoga is tuning into your body and discovering what it's telling you—however subtly—from one day to the next.

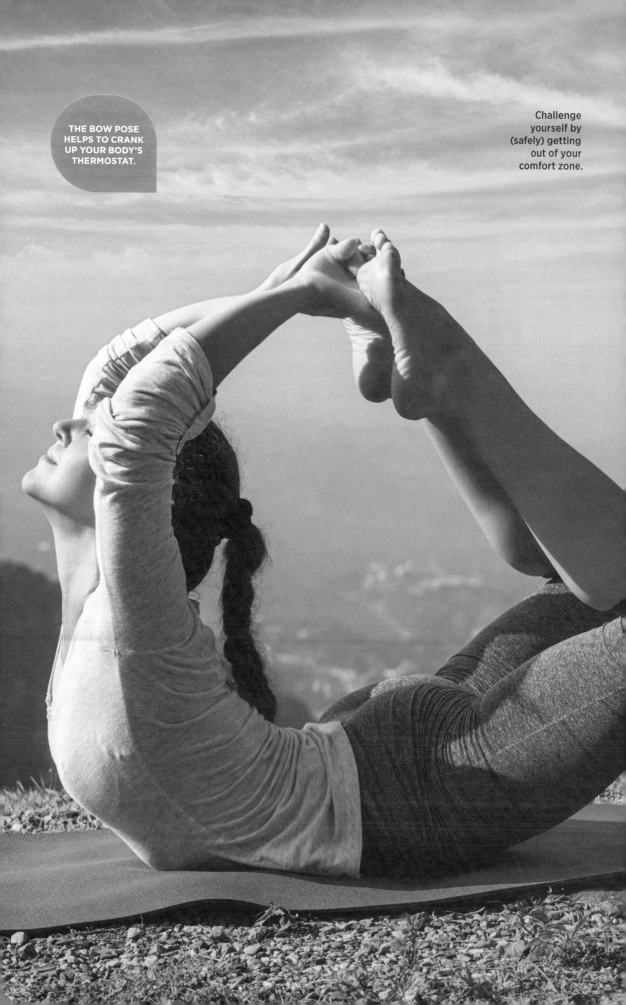

THE BOW POSE HELPS TO CRANK UP YOUR BODY'S THERMOSTAT.

Challenge yourself by (safely) getting out of your comfort zone.

BURN FAT AND GET FIT ON THE MAT

MOVING QUICKLY BETWEEN POSES WHILE ENGAGING ALL YOUR MAJOR MUSCLE GROUPS HELPS TO QUICKLY FIRE UP YOUR METABOLISM WHILE BLASTING FLAB.

Think yoga is all about sitting around and chanting "om" to get your zen on? Try again! Yogis across the globe tend to have light and agile bodies because yoga, especially the dynamic sequences we bring you in this workout, can increase the heart rate while also working the muscles deeply. That's one of the best ways to burn fat while toning muscle. This circuit is designed to guide you into higher and more challenging variations to ensure you're never "slacking off." This workout is about hard work! Luckily you do get to relax at the end.

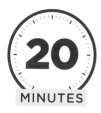

20
MINUTES

HOW TO DO IT
FAT-BURNING SERIES

Begin with one to two cycles of Sun Salutation (pages 52-53) to warm up. Then move to the floor to complete the following poses in the order they appear. Come onto all fours and rest as needed. If you have extra time, complete the full series twice through.

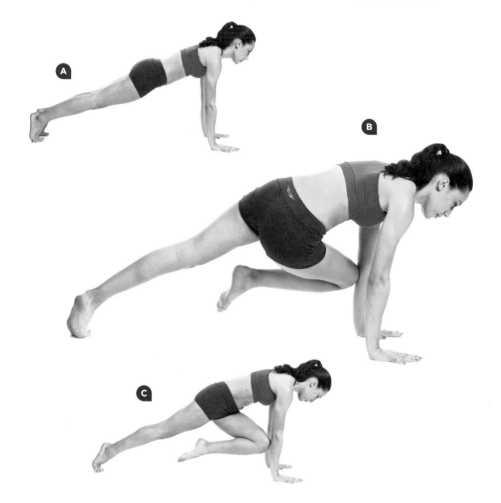

TWISTING PLANK POSE

1 Start on all fours, with hands shoulder-width apart directly under shoulders **(not shown)**.
2 Inhale, tuck your toes under and straighten your legs so you're in one line from your head sloping down to your feet **(A)**.
3 Exhale and tuck your chin in slightly. Keep the

back of your neck long and make a line from head to spine.
4 Engage abdominals, drawing them toward your spine. Keep breathing even and long.
5 Round your upper back to broaden your back and spread your shoulder blades apart.

6 Root palms into the floor with fingers fanned, elbows straight but not locked.
7 On an inhalation, engaging your belly and keeping your Plank stance, bring your right knee up and under your body toward your left elbow. Twist your body but make sure you keep your Plank

steady and your core squeezed **(B)**.
8 Repeat with left leg bent and left knee coming to right elbow **(C)**.
9 Do five to 10 alternating moves. Rest and repeat. Start with five alternating moves and build from there.

DOWNWARD-FACING DOG SPLITS AND HEAD-TO-KNEE SEQUENCE

1 Kneel on all fours, with legs hip-width apart, hands under your shoulders and your fingers fanning out **(not shown)**.

2 Exhale and curl your toes under and straighten your arms to lift your upper body while extending your legs to lift your hips up.

3 Draw your shoulder blades back and relax your head.

4 Draw in your abdominals, pull up your thigh muscles and stretch your heels back.

5 Straighten your legs—beginners or those with tight hamstrings can keep them bent. Point your tailbone to the ceiling **(A)**.

6 Point your heels back toward the floor. Focus on lengthening your legs and lifting your tailbone.

7 Now inhale and bring your right leg straight up behind you, pointing the toes **(B)**.

8 Exhale and bend your right knee, bringing it toward your right elbow. Bring your head down to meet it, as if you're going to kiss your knee **(C)**. Inhale as you stretch your leg out.

9 Repeat five to 10 times on each side.

10 Rest for a couple of breaths and repeat.

MAKE SURE YOU DON'T STRAIN YOUR NECK. THE POINT IS TO CREATE HEAT IN YOUR BODY.

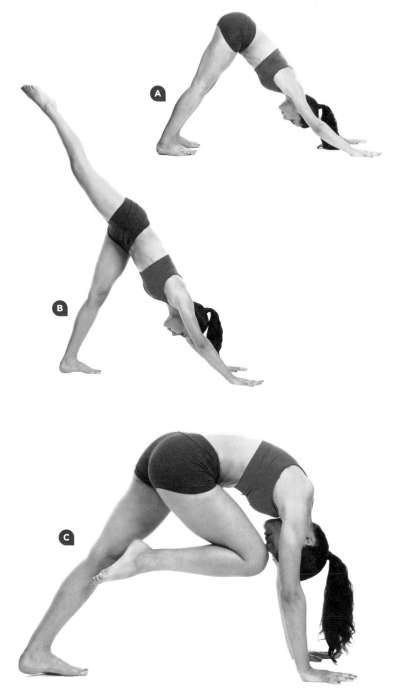

DYNAMIC BOAT POSE

BEGINNER VERSION

1 Sit on the floor with your legs straight out in front of you. On an inhalation, lift your feet off the floor a few inches. Hold the backs of your thighs for support. Engage your abdominals and move your torso diagonally back so you balance on your tailbone **(not shown)**.

2 Lift your feet, keeping your knees bent about 90 degrees and your shins parallel to the floor. Let go of your thighs if you can. Continue to balance on your tailbone **(A)**.

3 On an exhalation, lower your torso back until you're a few inches from the floor; straighten legs out **(B)**. Move back up to A. Repeat this in-out movement 10 times (going in and out equals one rep). If you need to, hold onto your thighs to rest between reps.

INTERMEDIATE VERSION

Do the move as above, but this time straighten your legs in front of you so your torso and legs are at a 45 degree angle, toes gently pointing up, feet relaxed and abs engaged. **(C)**

> TO BALANCE ON YOUR TAILBONE, SQUEEZE YOUR ABDOMINAL MUSCLES FOR SUPPORT.

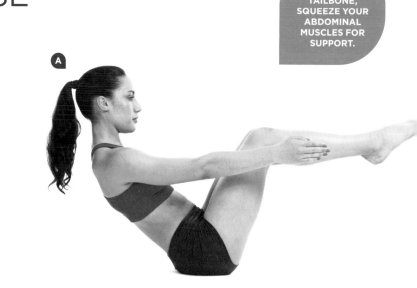

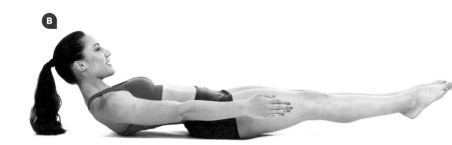

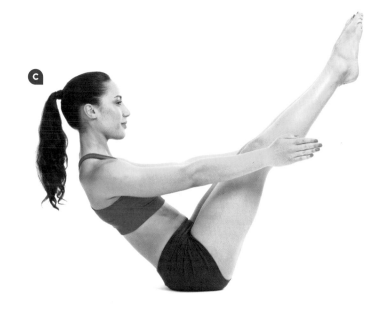

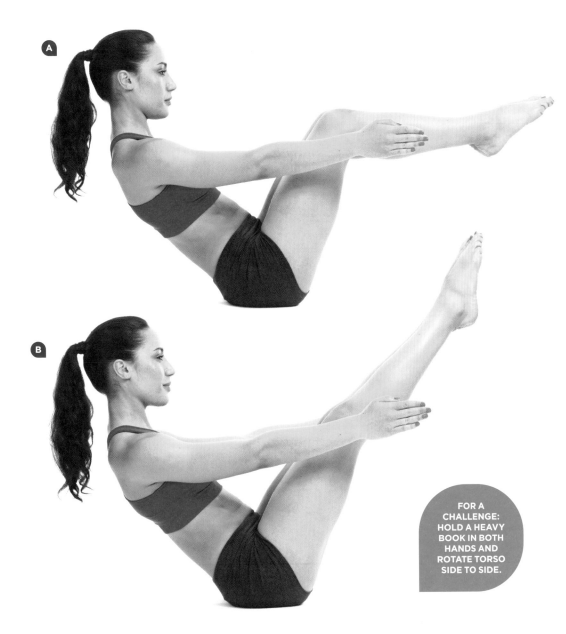

BOAT POSE

NAVASANA

1 Sit on the floor with your legs straight out in front of you. On an inhalation, lift your feet off the floor a few inches. Hold the backs of your thighs for support if necessary. Engage your abs and move torso diagonally back so you balance on your tailbone. This is stage one of the posture.

Take five breaths here, then rest and repeat.
2 Lift your feet and keep your knees bent so your shins are parallel to the floor and knees are bent 90 degrees. Continue to balance on your tailbone (A). Beginners stay in this pose for five breaths.

3 On an exhalation, lean back and straighten legs until the body is in a V-shape (B). Take five breaths. Rest and repeat.
4 Try squeezing a cushion or block between your inner thighs as you hold the pose.
5 Repeat Dynamic Boat Pose and this pose.

IMAGINE THE TOP OF YOUR HEAD AND YOUR FEET BEING PULLED IN OPPOSITE DIRECTIONS.

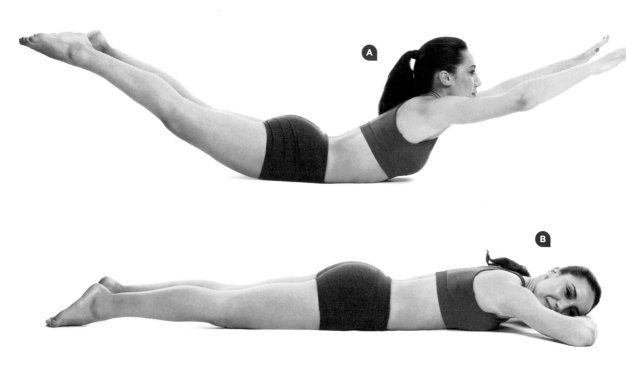

LOCUST

SALABHASANA

1 Lie facedown with your chin resting on the mat, feet facing down, arms above head, palms facing down. Take a few centering breaths **(1-4 not shown)**.
2 Inhale and lift one leg up, firm it, turn it inward,

stretch it back and exhale to lower it. Do this with the other leg.
3 Keeping the muscles on your legs firm, draw your tailbone toward your heels and press your pubic bone into the mat.

4 Inhale and, keeping your neck long, lift both thighs, your head and chest away from the floor.
5 Stretch your arms out in front of you and lift them as you raise your legs and feet **(A)**.

6 Take three to five breaths and release on an exhalation, lowering your arms and legs. Put one hand over the other and rest your head to one side **(B)**.

BOW

DHANURASANA

1 Lie facedown with forehead resting on hands **(A)**.
2 Bend knees so shins are perpendicular to floor. Inhale, extend right arm toward feet. Exhale and release. Repeat with other hand.
3 Inhale and extend both arms toward your feet, taking hold of your ankles or shins **(B)**. Exhale.

4 Inhale and press the front of your feet into your hands while lifting your heels from your buttocks toward the ceiling, then lift your thighs off the floor. This should open your chest and lift your head and chest off the floor.
5 Press your tailbone and pubic bone into the mat. Draw your shoulders down

and open and lift your chest further, pointing your sternum upward **(C)**.
6 Keeping your breath steady, focus on bringing your knees, ankles and feet closer so you feel an opening in your entire body. Take five to 10 breaths.
7 Repeat three to five times, resting for a few seconds in between.

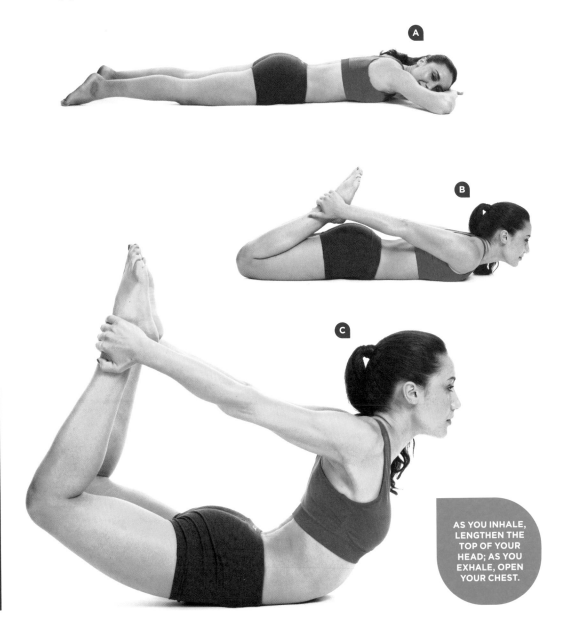

AS YOU INHALE, LENGTHEN THE TOP OF YOUR HEAD; AS YOU EXHALE, OPEN YOUR CHEST.

PIGEON POSE

EKA PADA RAJAKAPOTASANA

KEEP YOUR BACK LEG FACING DOWN AND YOUR WEIGHT EVENLY DISTRIBUTED.

1 Start on all fours with your knees beneath your hips and your hands beneath your shoulders **(A)**.

2 Lift your left knee and place it a few inches behind your left wrist.

3 Gently slide back your right leg, straightening it.

4 Place your left heel in front of your right hip. As you progress in this pose, move the heel of your bent leg further away from the front of your hip to help open your hips.

5 Inhale and lengthen your torso by extending your crown to the ceiling, pressing your fingers into the floor, straightening your arms and drawing your chin to your chest **(B)**. Exhale. Ensure your weight is even on both hips.

6 Inhale, move your torso forward, root your palms and forearms to the floor and lift your chest, drawing back your shoulder blades. Look ahead and take five to 10 deep breaths **(C)**.

7 On an exhalation, lean your torso over your bent leg and relax down—use a bolster if you can't reach the floor. Rest your forehead on your hands. Take another five to 10 breaths **(D)**.

8 Release the pose by pressing your hands into the floor, lifting your hips and moving back to your hands and knees. Repeat on the other side.

VARIATION If you have tight hips and your bent-leg hip is lifting off the floor, place a block or folded blanket under it for support.

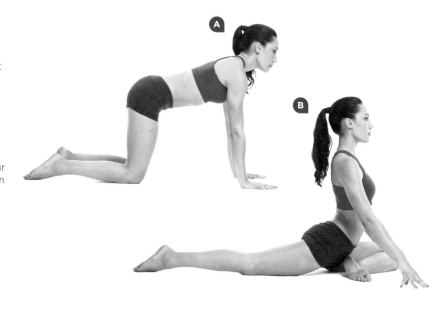

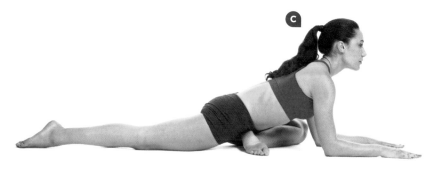

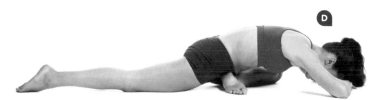

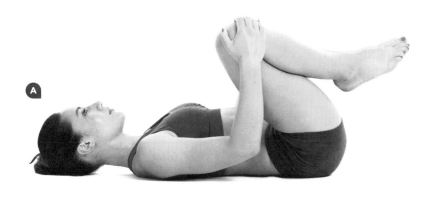

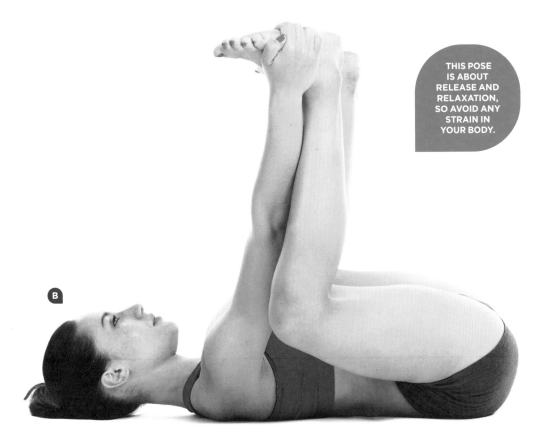

HAPPY BABY

ANANDA BALASANA

1 Begin by lying on your back. Bend both knees deeply, slightly wider than your body **(A)**.
2 Flex your feet and take your outer feet with your hands.
3 Bend your knees toward your armpits. Feel the stretch and deep release in your lower back.
4 Draw your chin slightly in to lengthen your neck, keep your shoulders down and relaxed and point your tailbone forward to lengthen your spine **(B)**.

5 Take 10 to 20 breaths, rocking from side to side if it feels comfortable, then release your feet to the floor.

VARIATION If you can't easily hold your feet, grasp the back of your shins.

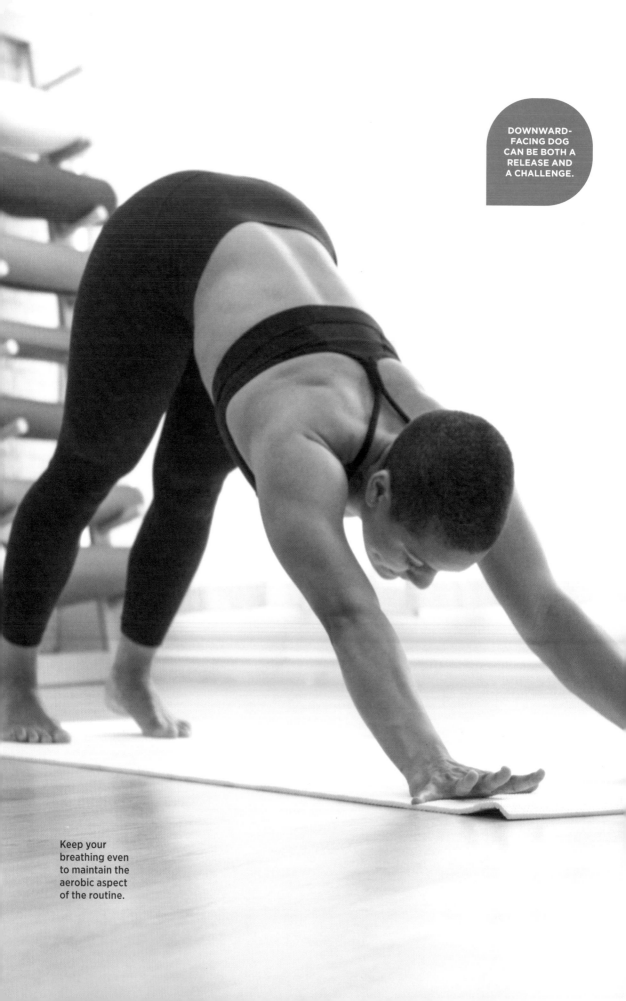

DOWNWARD-FACING DOG CAN BE BOTH A RELEASE AND A CHALLENGE.

Keep your breathing even to maintain the aerobic aspect of the routine.

YOGA CARDIO YOU'LL LOVE

GET YOUR HEART RATE SOARING WITH A SEQUENCE OF POSES THAT BLASTS CALORIES, BOOSTS METABOLISM AND SCULPTS MUSCLES FROM HEAD TO TOE.

You don't need to run miles or spin endlessly to work up a sweat and raise your heart rate. Yoga, when practiced with a series of flowing poses, can be a powerful way to build cardiovascular fitness. To maximize results, keep your breathing consistent while holding the postures and jump your legs as you switch sides. This routine builds by adding poses throughout the series, allowing repetition for improving alignment and stamina. This is followed by slowing the heart rate down with deep hip openers and a core-strengthening sequence.

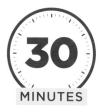

30 MINUTES

HOW TO DO IT
AEROBIC BOOSTER

This 30-minute sequence can seem a bit complicated at first but you'll soon get the hang of it. You'll repeat some poses (like the Low Lunge and High Lunge) several times. To get your heart rate up, jump your legs back and forth as you switch sides; if you need to take it easier, just step each foot forward and back. Find a map of the full series on pages 84-85.

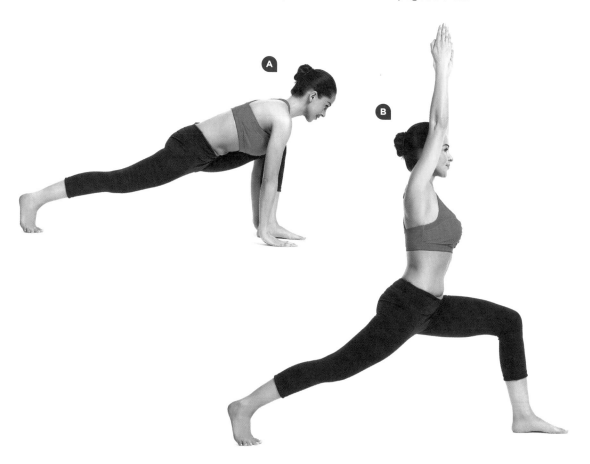

LOW LUNGE & HIGH LUNGE
ASHVA SANCHALANASANA & ALANASANA

1 Begin with a few rounds of the Sun Salutation series on pages 52-53. Then get into a high push-up, hands on floor below shoulders, legs extended **(not shown)**.
2 Exhale and bring left foot forward between hands. Bend left knee 90 degrees, aligning knee directly over

left heel. Keep both feet facing forward and hip-width apart and hands flat on the mat, fingers spread. Straighten right leg and tuck toes under. Draw right hip forward as you press left hip back, keeping hips parallel to top edge of mat **(A)**. Stay here for five breaths.

3 Inhale and stretch arms overhead, keeping left knee bent. Sink hips and pelvis downward **(B)**.
4 Point the heel of your right foot behind you, putting weight into straight right leg. Relax shoulders, look straight ahead and take five full breaths.

5 Return to Low Lunge. Jump feet, switching legs three times. Land with right foot forward. Repeat Low Lunge/High Lunge sequence with right foot forward, holding both poses for five breaths. Jump feet, switching legs three times to finish with left foot forward.

WARRIOR II & REVERSE WARRIOR

VIRABHADRASANA II & VIPARITA VIRABHADRASANA

1 From Low Lunge with left foot forward, move to High Lunge. Lower right foot to mat, turning it so the heel of your left foot is in line with the arch of your right foot. Place hands on hips **(A)**.

2 Inhale and extend your arms out parallel to the floor, palms down. Extend your fingers and keep your shoulders soft. Lengthen your tailbone down and straighten your torso so your don't overarch your back.

3 Exhale, and bend left knee 90 degrees, shin perpendicular to floor. Lift your inner arches, rooting the outer edges of your feet; engage the muscles in your back leg. Turn your head to gaze over left arm. Hold for five breaths **(B)**.

4 Return to Low Lunge and jump, switching legs three times. Repeat Warrior II on opposite side. Place hands on floor for Low Lunge and jump legs three times, so left foot is forward; return to Warrior II with arms extended at shoulder height.

5 Raise your left arm over your head and lean back over your straight right leg. Root down into your feet **(C)**.

6 Hold for three to five deep breaths. Inhale and return to Warrior II. Then move directly into Extended Side Angle (see page 74).

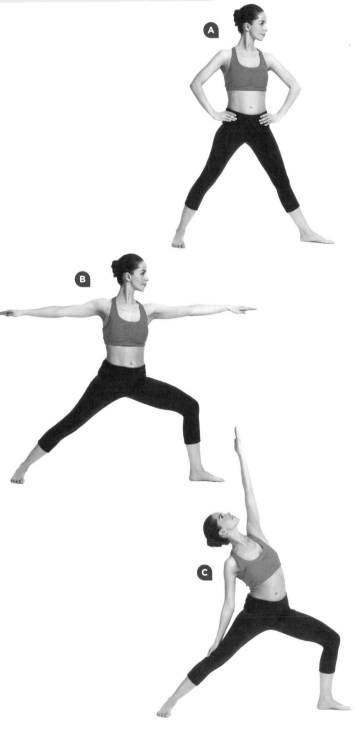

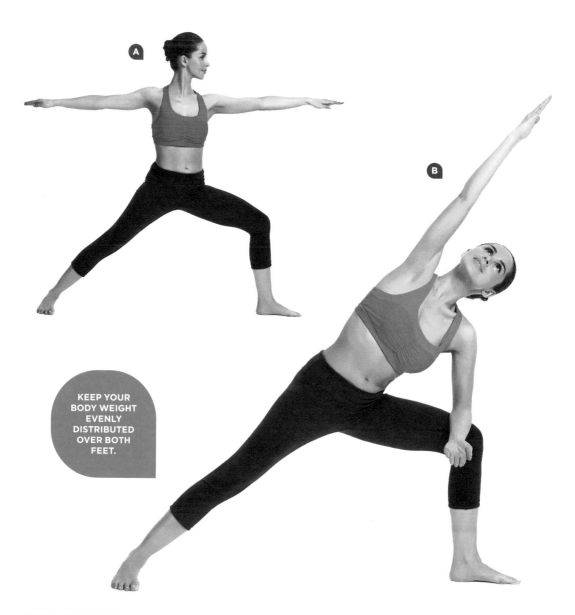

KEEP YOUR BODY WEIGHT EVENLY DISTRIBUTED OVER BOTH FEET.

EXTENDED SIDE ANGLE

UTTHITA PARSVAKONASANA

1 From Warrior II **(A)**, inhale and extend your torso over your left thigh without bending your body forward or lifting your feet. 2 Place your left forearm on your left thigh for support. Exhale and extend your right arm over your head and look up to your right hand **(B)**. Hold here for three to five breaths, pressing down into the outer edge of your left foot and engaging your core. Move directly into Half Moon (see page 75), keeping your left leg forward.

HALF MOON

ARDHA CHANDRASANA

1 From Extended Side Angle, place a block about a foot in front of your left foot. Inhale and extend your right arm to the ceiling, bend your left leg and slide your right foot toward your left foot. Place your left hand on the block **(A)**.

2 Raise your right leg to the side, parallel to the floor. Keeping your right foot flexed and facing forward, turn your head to look up toward your right hand—if this strains your neck, keep looking straight ahead **(B)**. Hold here for five breaths. Boost your balance by contracting your abdominals and supporting leg, and pointing your right ankle toward the back of the room.

3 To release, bend your left leg slightly before lowering the right leg to the floor.

4 Step back to Warrior II, then place hands down to Low Lunge. Jump and switch legs three times.

5 Repeat sequence on opposite side (right foot forward), flowing from Low Lunge to High Lunge to Warrior II to Reverse Warrior to Extended Side Angle to Half Moon. Step back into Warrior II. Place hands on floor for Low Lunge with right foot forward, then place both knees on floor so you are down on all fours. Move into Downward-Facing Dog (see page 76).

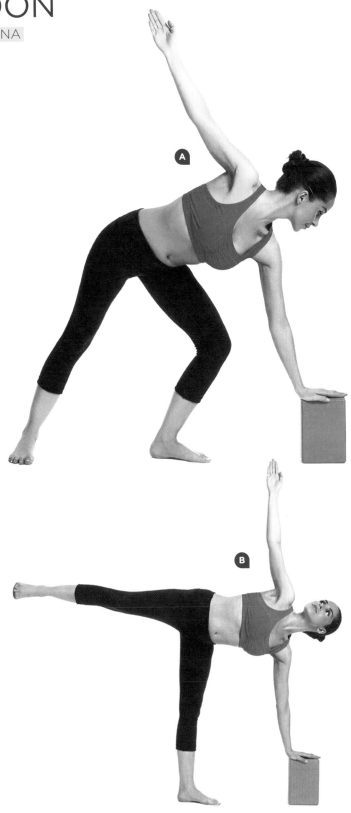

DOWNWARD-FACING DOG

ADHO MUKHA SVANASANA

1 Begin on all fours with your legs hip-width apart, hands under your shoulders and your fingers fanning out. Inhale.

2 Exhale and curl your toes under, straighten your arms and extend your legs to raise your hips up toward the ceiling.

3 Draw your shoulders back and relax your head.

4 Draw in your abs, press your thighs back and extend your heels toward the back of the room.

5 Straighten your legs as much as possible, pointing tailbone to the ceiling. Extend your heels to the floor but don't worry if they don't reach.

6 Focus on flattening your back, keeping your shoulder blades pulled back and looking toward your knees. Keep your thigh muscles strong.

7 Root your hands into the floor and take six to 10 deep breaths before moving into Three-Legged Downward-Facing Dog (see page 77).

> **REACH YOUR TAILBONE UP WHILE PRESSING YOUR HANDS AND FEET INTO THE FLOOR.**

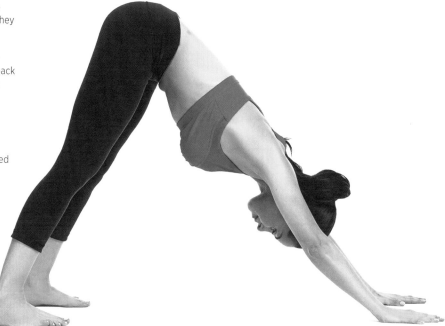

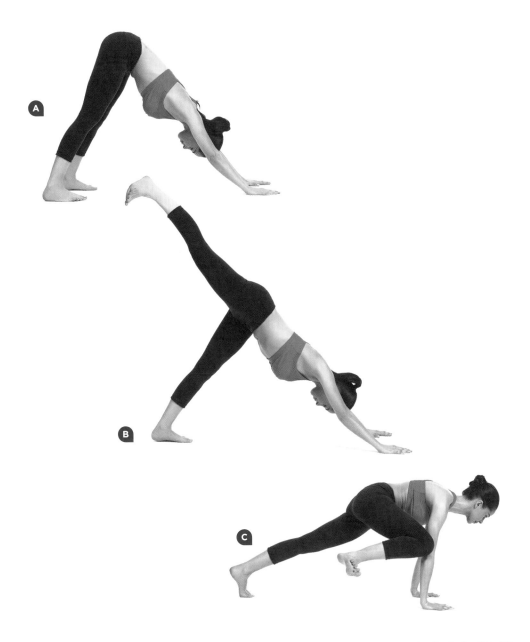

THREE-LEGGED DOWNWARD-FACING DOG WITH VARIATION
TRI PADA ADHO MUKHA SVANASANA

1 From Downward-Facing Dog **(A)**, inhale and bring your right leg straight up behind you and flex your foot **(B)**.
2 Keep your hips squared to the floor and hold for three breaths, pressing your left foot into the floor.
3 Lower your right leg and bring in toward your right elbow, keeping right foot lifted **(C)**.
4 Lift right leg back up behind you, then lower it across your body toward left elbow **(not shown)**. Return to Three-Legged Downward-Facing Dog and repeat knee to same elbow and knee to opposite elbow three times. Lower right foot to Downward-Facing Dog.
5 Repeat sequence, this time lifting left leg. Finish back in Downward-Facing Dog, then return to all fours to move into Plank (see page 78).

KEEP YOUR ABS FIRM AND YOUR HEAD IN LINE WITH YOUR SPINE.

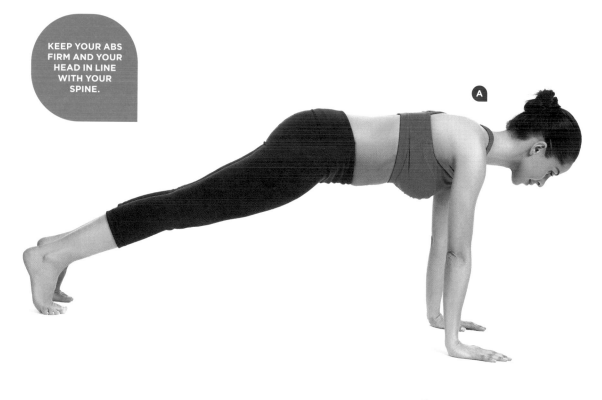

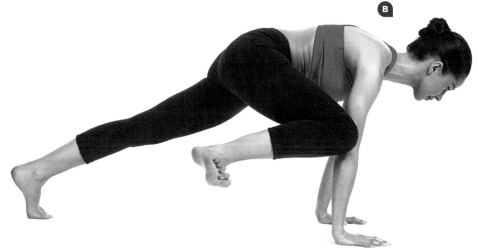

PLANK WITH VARIATION
KUMBHAKASANA

1 Begin on all fours, hands shoulder-width apart and directly under shoulders. Inhale, tucking toes under and straightening your legs so you're in a diagonal line from your head to your feet.
2 Exhale, and tuck your chin in slightly, keeping back of your neck long. Engage your abdominal muscles, drawing them toward your spine **(A)**.
3 Inhale and bring right knee to the outside of your right arm, touching your elbow **(B)**. Pause, then exhale and return right leg to Plank. Hold five breaths, then bring left knee to the outside of left elbow. Return to Plank, then get back on all fours for Pigeon Pose (page 79).

PIGEON

EKA PADA RAJAKAPOTASANA PREP

1 Start on all fours with your knees beneath your hips and your hands beneath your shoulders **(A)**.

2 Lift your left knee and place it a few inches behind your right wrist. Slide your right leg back, straightening it out.

3 Place your left heel in front of your right hip. As you progress, move the heel of your bent leg further from the front of your hip to open your hips.

4 Inhale, and lengthen torso by extending crown of head to the ceiling, pressing your fingers into the floor and chin to chest **(B)**.

5 Exhale, lean torso over bent leg and relax down. Use a bolster if you can't reach the floor. Stay here for a few deep breaths **(C)**. Keep weight even on both hips; try not to tilt to one side. On an inhale, press palms into the floor and lift your torso, drawing tailbone down and core up, pressing your hips into the mat. Exhale.

6 Release by pressing hands into the floor, lifting hips and moving back onto hands and knees. Repeat on the other side, finishing on all fours before moving into Locust (see page 80).

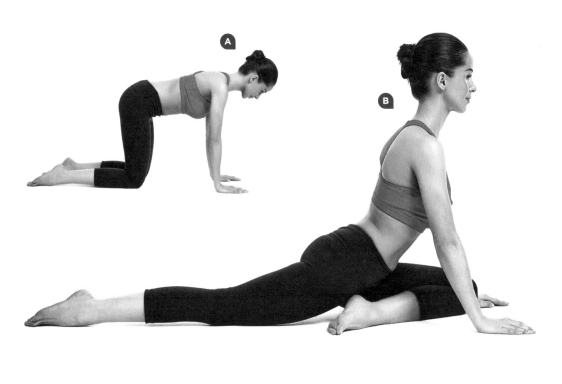

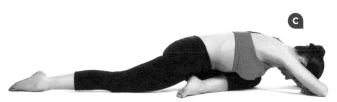

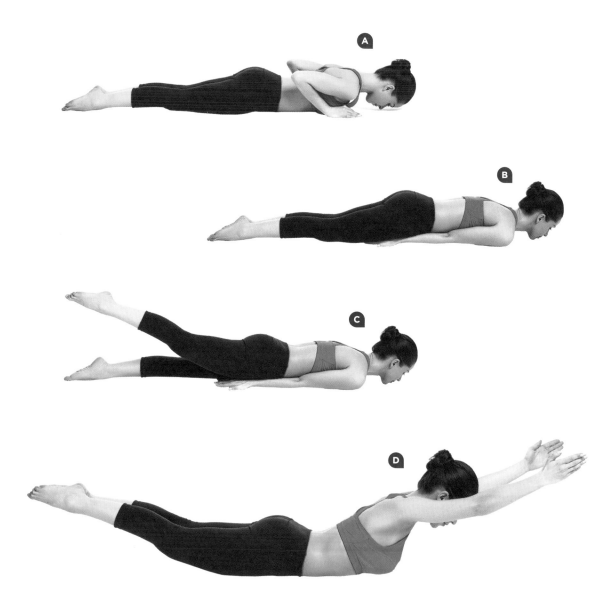

LOCUST

SALABHASANA

1 From all fours, lie facedown with forehead resting on the floor, hands beneath shoulders, elbows tucked into sides **(A)**. Turn your big toes toward each other to inwardly rotate your thighs.
2 Lifting your right hip, straighten your right arm and tuck it under your hip

and torso. Do the same with your left arm **(B)**.
3 Keeping your toes pointing backward, exhale and slowly lift your right leg off the floor. Firm your buttocks, and reach strongly through your leg **(C)**. Hold for five breaths, lower leg, then repeat on other side.

4 Exhale and lift your head, upper torso, arms and legs away from the floor. Firm your buttocks and look down at the floor. You'll be resting on your lower ribs, belly and front pelvis. Bring your arms forward in line with your ears, palms facing inward **(D)**. Keep your big toes turned toward each

other and reach strongly through your legs. Take five to 10 breaths then release with an exhalation, lowering back to floor to prepare for Bow (see page 81).

BOW

DHANURASANA

1 Lie facedown with your hands alongside your torso, palms up. Exhale and bend your knees, bringing your feet as close to your bottom as you can. Reach back with your hands and take hold of your ankles—but not the tops of your feet. Look down at the floor **(A)**. Keep your knees hip-width apart.
2 Inhale, and as you exhale, strongly lift your heels away from your buttocks and lift your thighs away from the floor. Push your tailbone toward the floor, keep your back muscles soft and look straight ahead **(B)**.
3 Draw the tops of your shoulders away from ears and press shoulder blades down. Take five to 10 breaths. Release as you exhale. Stay here for a breath, then roll over so you are faceup, ready to move into Supine Spinal Twist (see page 82).

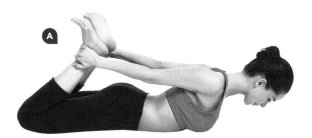

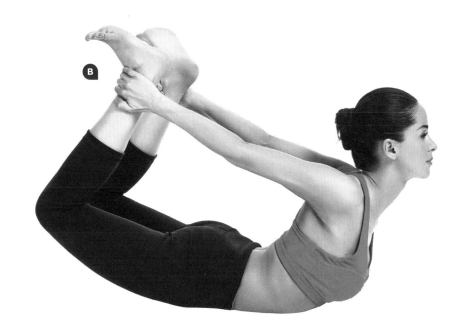

DON'T BE SURPRISED IF ONE SIDE IS TIGHTER THAN THE OTHER—GO ONLY AS FAR AS YOU CAN.

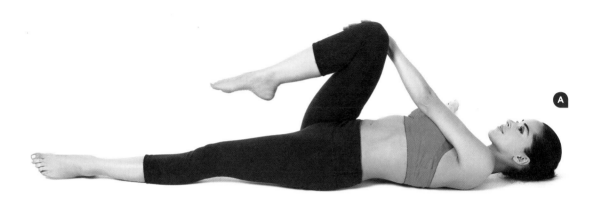

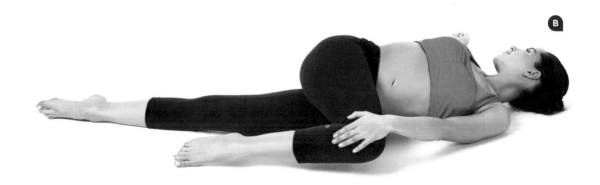

SUPINE SPINAL TWIST

SUPTA MATSYENDRASANA

1 Lie faceup on the floor. Bend your right knee. Exhale and take your right knee with your left hand, guiding your right leg over to your left. Bring right arm out to right side, perpendicular to torso. **(A)**.

2 Exhale and rotate further, bringing your right knee down to the floor as far as you comfortably can. Turn your head to the right **(B)**.

3 Hold for several breaths.

4 Inhale and release back to the start position.

5 Repeat on the other side. Lower both legs back so you are faceup on floor for the Corpse (see page 83).

USE THIS POSE DURING YOUR PRACTICE TO RECOVER FROM A CHALLENGING SEQUENCE.

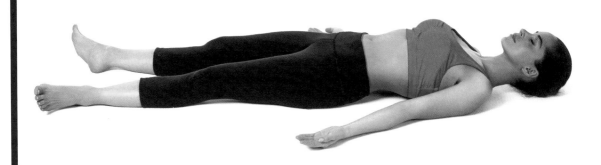

CORPSE

SAVASANA

1 Lie faceup on floor with your feet hip-width apart.
2 Turn your palms to face the ceiling with your arms relaxed and about a foot away from your body.

3 Relax hands, allowing fingers to gently curl.
4 Slide shoulders down and relax your neck.
5 Straighten legs and let your feet fall to the sides.

6 Close your eyes, relax your body and breath and let go. Stay here about three to five minutes, or as long as you feel is necessary, breathing evenly and slowly, completing this aerobic sequence.

CARDIO FLOW SEQUENCE

Warm-up sequence (Sun Salutation; see pages 52-53) to High Push-Up **(not shown)**.

1 Low Lunge (see page 72).
2 High Lunge (see page 72). Hold both poses for five breaths, then from Low Lunge, jump legs three times to land with right foot forward. Repeat Low Lunge to High Lunge on right side; hold both poses for five breaths.
3 Jump legs three times, finishing in Low Lunge with left foot forward.
4 Return to High Lunge.
5 Warrior II (see page 73); hold for five breaths. Return to Low Lunge. Jump legs three times to land with right foot forward. Repeat Warrior II with right foot forward.
6 Return to Low Lunge and jump legs three times so left foot is forward.
7 Move into High Lunge, keeping left foot forward.
8 Warrior II, left foot forward.
9 Reverse Warrior (see page 73). Hold for three breaths.
10 Extended Side Angle (see page 74). Hold for three breaths.
11 Half Moon (see page 75); hold for five breaths.
12 Step back to Warrrior II.
13 Place hands down into Low Lunge. Jump and switch legs three times. Repeat on right side, from Warrior II to Reverse Warrior to Extended Side Angle to Half Moon to Warrior II to Low Lunge.
14 Downward-Facing Dog (see page 76); hold for six to 10 breaths
15 Three-Legged Downward-Facing Dog (see page 77), right leg lifted. Hold for three breaths.

16 Right knee to right elbow (see page 77).
17 Three-Legged Downward-Facing Dog; knee crosses to opposite elbow **(not shown)**; return to Three-Legged Downward-Facing Dog. Repeat three times. Stop at Downward-Facing Dog. Repeat with left leg.
18 Plank (see page 78).
19 Right knee to right elbow. Return to Plank. Hold for five breaths, then left knee to left elbow; return to Plank.
20 Pigeon (see page 79) with left knee bent for five breaths. Repeat on opposite side.
21 Locust (see page 80) for five to 10 breaths.
22 Bow (see page 81) for five to 10 breaths.
23 Supine Spinal Twist (see page 82) with right knee bent. Switch sides and repeat.
24 Corpse (see page 83). Hold for three to five minutes.

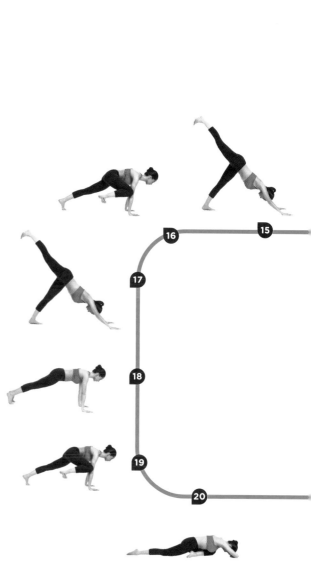

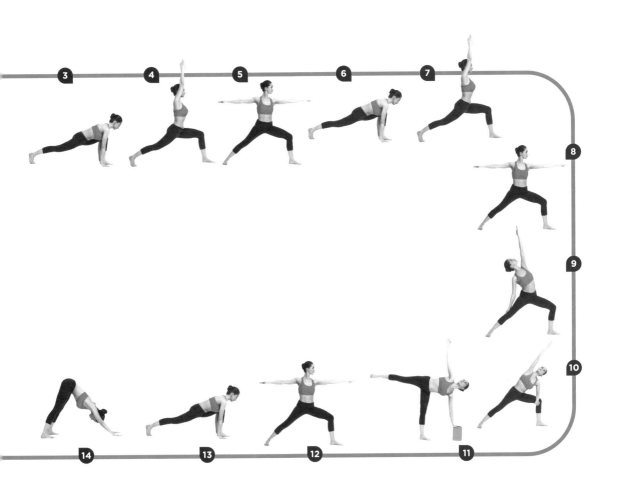

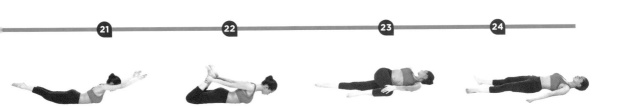

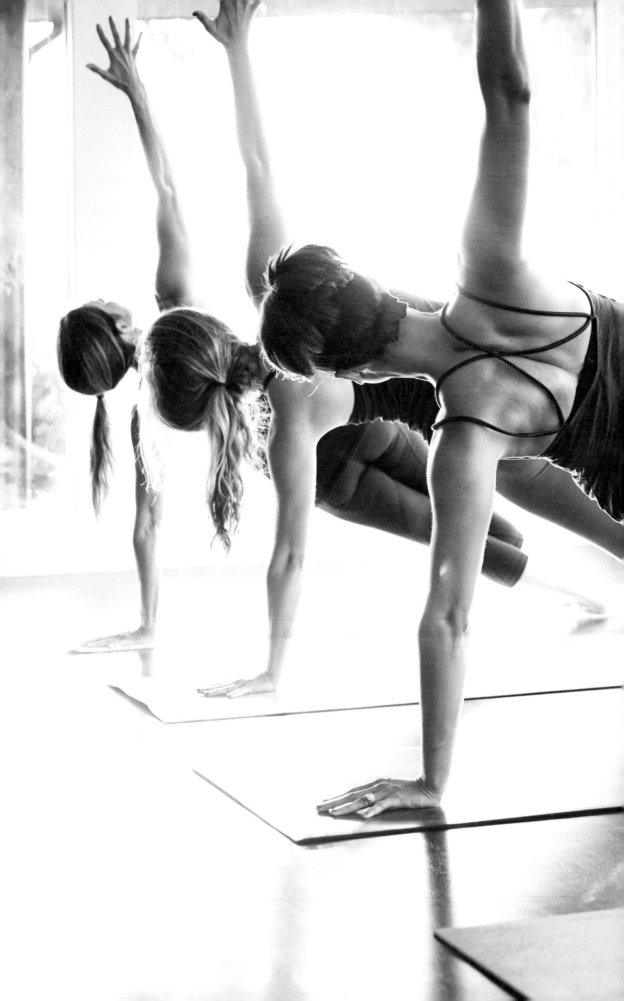

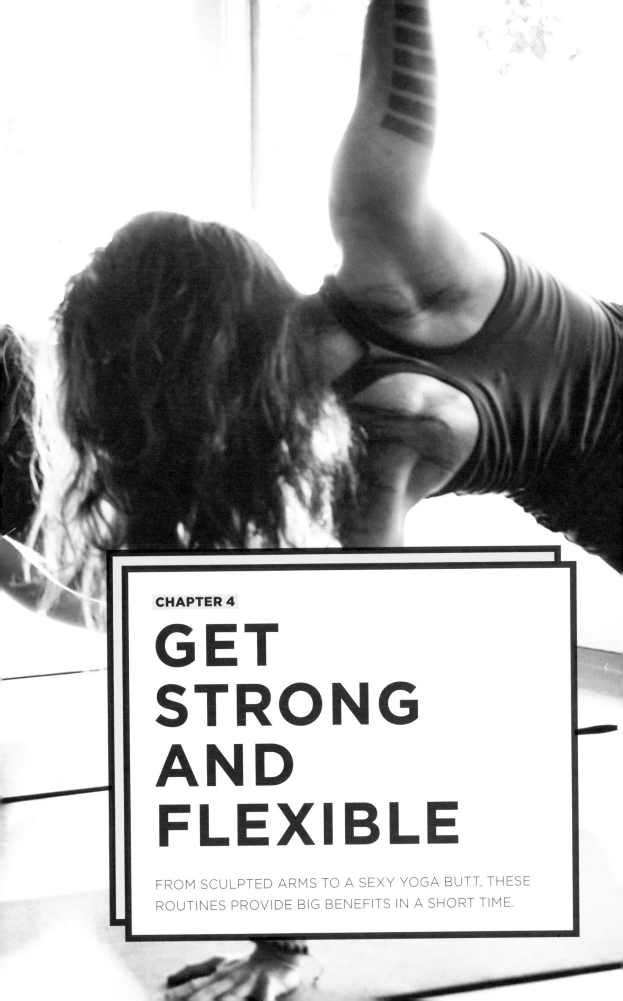

CHAPTER 4

GET STRONG AND FLEXIBLE

FROM SCULPTED ARMS TO A SEXY YOGA BUTT, THESE ROUTINES PROVIDE BIG BENEFITS IN A SHORT TIME.

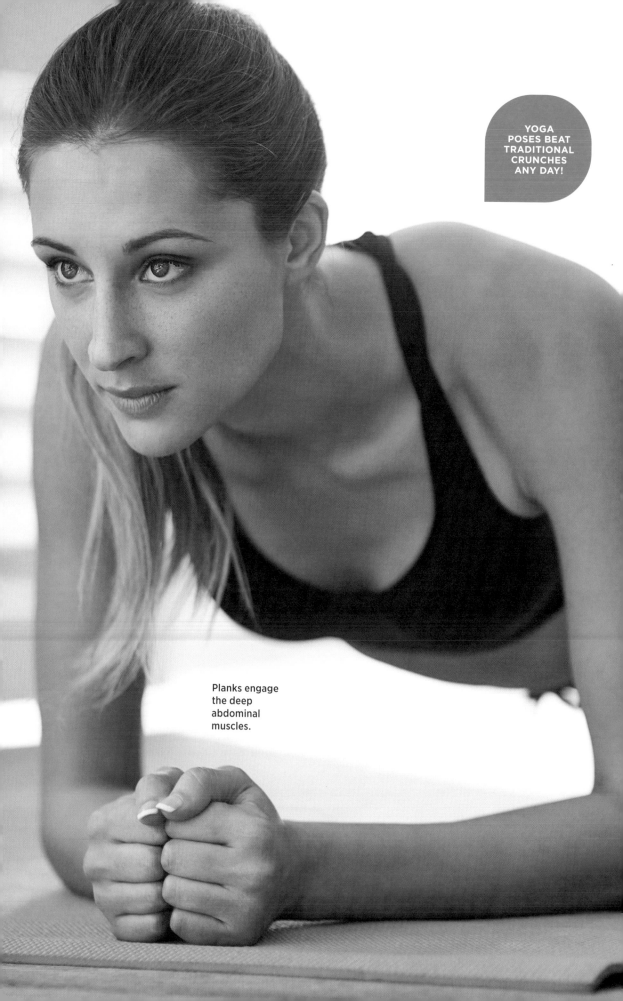

Planks engage the deep abdominal muscles.

TONE AND TIGHTEN YOUR CORE

ALMOST EVERY YOGA POSTURE INVOLVES THE ABDOMINALS TO SOME DEGREE—BUT THESE HAVE AN EXTRA FOCUS ON SCULPTING YOUR SIX PACK AND MORE.

Your core muscles are not only about having strong, defined abs—although who doesn't want those? In yoga, the core relates to the entire "corset" of muscle (front, back and sides) between your ribs and groin. This workout will challenge this area, especially the oblique muscles at the outer edges of your core, which rarely get used. Some poses will challenge you, so start small and build from there. It's not just about aesthetics—a strong core looks great, but it also helps prevent back pain, as these muscles are key to supporting your spine and keeping you upright.

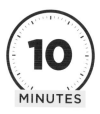

10 MINUTES

HOW TO DO IT
FIRM YOUR ABS

Sculpt your entire core—abs, obliques and lower back—with this series of seated and standing moves that will work the muscles from a variety of angles. Do them in the order given. If time permits, complete the sequence twice through, modifying as needed.

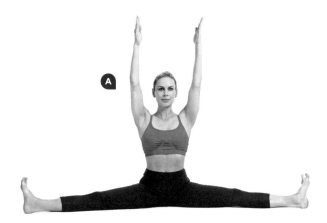

A

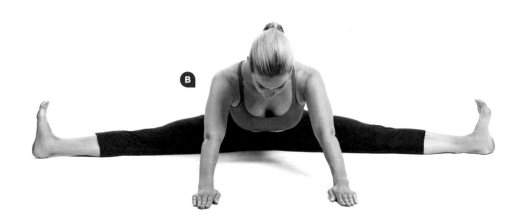

B

WIDE-ANGLE SEATED FORWARD BEND

UPAVISTHA KONASANA

1 Sit with legs wide apart in a V-shape (or wider if your flexibility allows).
2 Inhale and draw your arms over your head, keeping shoulders down, rooting pelvis down and lengthening spine **(A)**.

3 Exhale and tilt forward from hips, keeping spine straight and knees facing up. Place your hands flat on the floor in front, shoulder-width apart. Keep your neck long and chin slightly tucked in.

4 Keep your knees and toes pointing upward, heels extending forward, feet flexed and thigh muscles engaged and rooted. Don't rotate your legs inward or outward to come further forward **(B)**.

5 Take five to 10 deep breaths, extending your spine on each inhalation and releasing further into the stretch on exhalation.
6 Keep your feet flexed and pointing upward and your knees pointing upward.

SEATED WIDE-LEGGED SIDE STRETCH

1 Sit up tall with your legs in a V. Inhale and draw your arms up over your head, rooting your pelvis down and lengthening your spine upward **(A)**.
2 Exhale and stretch your torso sideways, taking your left big toe in your left hand or resting your hand or forearm (whatever is most comfortable) inside left knee or shin with your arm bent.
3 Inhale and extend your right arm out over your right ear, keeping your neck long and relaxed and your shoulders open. Rotate your right shoulder back and your left shoulder forward so they remain open. Feel the stretch down your right side **(B)**.
4 Keep the backs of your legs grounded to the floor with feet flexing upward.
5 Take eight deep breaths, feeling the deep stretch in your side. Repeat on the other side.

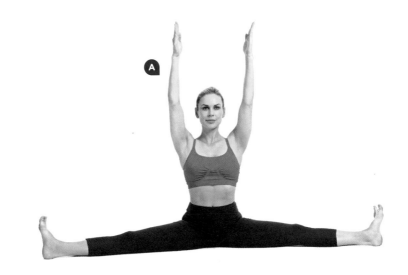

IF YOU CAN'T REACH YOUR TOES, HOLD ONTO YOUR ANKLE OR SHIN.

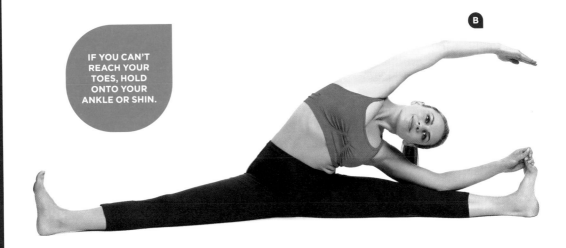

PLANK WITH TOE TAPS

1 Start on all fours with your hands shoulder-width apart directly under your shoulders.
2 Inhale, tuck your toes under and straighten your legs so you're in one diagonal line, from your head sloping down to your feet.

3 Exhale and tuck your chin in slightly, keep the back of your neck long and make a line from your head to your spine to form Plank **(A)**.
4 Engage your abdominal muscles, drawing them toward your spine. Keep breathing even and long—it's tempting to hold it!

5 Round your upper back to broaden your back and spread your shoulder blades apart.
6 Root your palms into the floor with your fingers fanning out, elbows straight but not locked.
7 Do five to 10 toe taps with left foot out to side **(B)**.

8 Repeat on the right foot.
9 Do two sets on each side, alternating with Side Plank (page 93).

VARIATION
If this is too hard, hold Plank and start with one to two taps then build up; engaging abs will help.

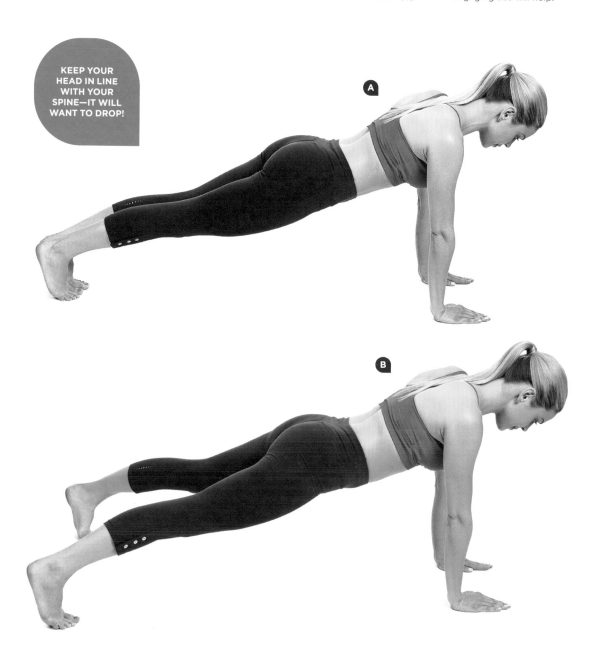

KEEP YOUR HEAD IN LINE WITH YOUR SPINE—IT WILL WANT TO DROP!

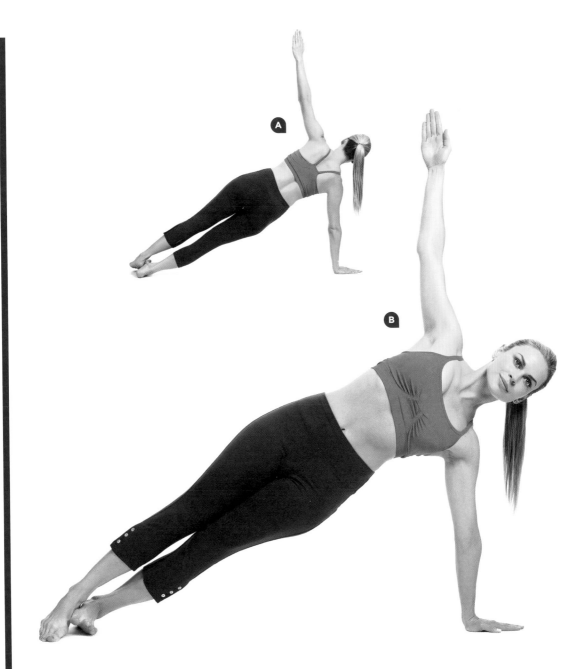

SIDE PLANK

VASISTHASANA

1 From Plank, inhale and press your right hand into the floor and roll over on to the outside edge of your right foot.
2 Exhale and stack your left ankle, hip and shoulder directly over your right ankle, hip and shoulder, balancing your body weight on your right hand and the outer edge of your right foot. Keep right arm directly under your right shoulder, pressing into the floor, drawing your abs toward your spine and keeping your hips lifted.
3 Inhale and lift your left arm up, open your chest and look straight ahead (A). Take five deep breaths, building up the length you hold the pose.
4 Repeat on the other side (B).

VARIATION To make it easier, bend top leg and place foot on the floor for support.

TREE POSE
BENDING AT WAIST

VRKSASANA

1 Stand tall with arms down at sides. Root your right foot into the floor and transfer your weight onto your right leg.
2 Lengthen your tailbone toward the floor and engage your belly. Exhale.
3 Inhale and place your left foot on your inner right thigh—or calf for beginners (not your knee). Exhale, pressing the sole of your left foot into your right thigh, turn your left knee out at 90 degrees, drawing your tailbone down **(A)**.
4 Keeping your shoulders relaxed and your chest lifted, inhale and lift your arms up over your head **(B)**.
5 Stretch both arms over to the left, keeping your body facing forward so you really feel the stretch along your right waistline **(C)**.
6 Take five to eight breaths. Repeat on the other side.

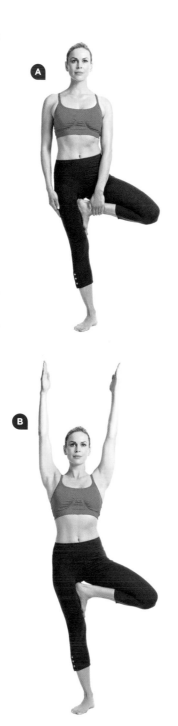

A

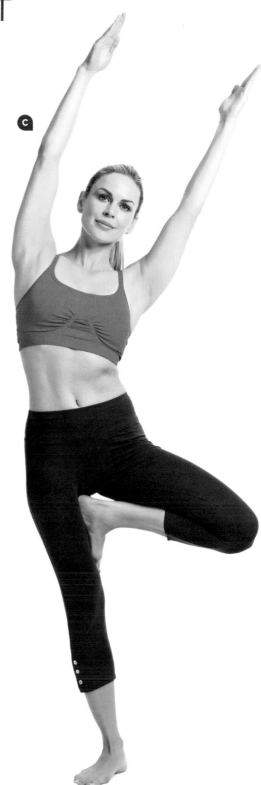

C

B

STAY STEADY BY FOCUSING ON A POINT ABOUT TWO YARDS IN FRONT OF YOU.

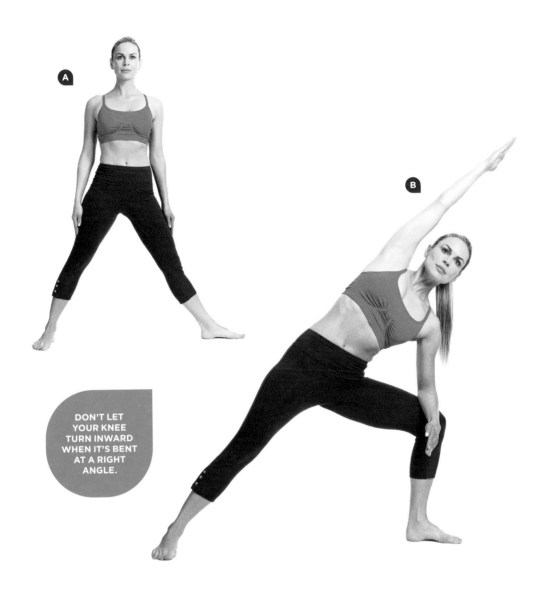

A

B

DON'T LET YOUR KNEE TURN INWARD WHEN IT'S BENT AT A RIGHT ANGLE.

EXTENDED SIDE ANGLE POSE

UTTHITA PARSVAKONASANA

1 Stand tall with arms down at sides. Step your feet a little more than a leg's-length distance apart, your left foot facing out and right foot turned slightly **(A)**.

2 On an in-breath, stretch your arms out to the sides, parallel to the floor, with your palms facing down.

3 Exhale and bend your left knee to a right angle, with your left knee directly over your left ankle.

4 Inhale and extend torso to the left over left thigh.

5 Place your left elbow on your left knee and lean your torso to the left.

6 Root into the outer edge

of your back foot. Ensure your torso stays strong and doesn't collapse, and lift your abdominals back toward your spine.

7 Extend your right arm over your head **(B)**. Keep your shoulders down and relaxed. Take a breath and press down into both feet to come up.

REVERSE WARRIOR

VIPARITA VIRABHADRASANA

1 From Extended Side Angle Pose (page 95), inhale and come up **(A)**, bringing your right hand down the back of your right leg and bending your left knee.

2 Bring your left arm up and over, arch your back and move your head toward your right leg—your left arm should be tracking next to your ear.

3 Keeping your front knee bent deeply, reach your rear hand down the leg as you come into a back bend.

4 Bring your gaze up to your fingertips but don't strain your neck or throw your head back **(B)**.

5 Your support should be coming from your legs and core, not your back hand.

6 Complete your inhalation and move back into the Extended Side Angle Pose. After the fifth time through with each pose, hold there for five breaths.

7 Repeat Extended Side Angle and Reverse Warrior on opposite side.

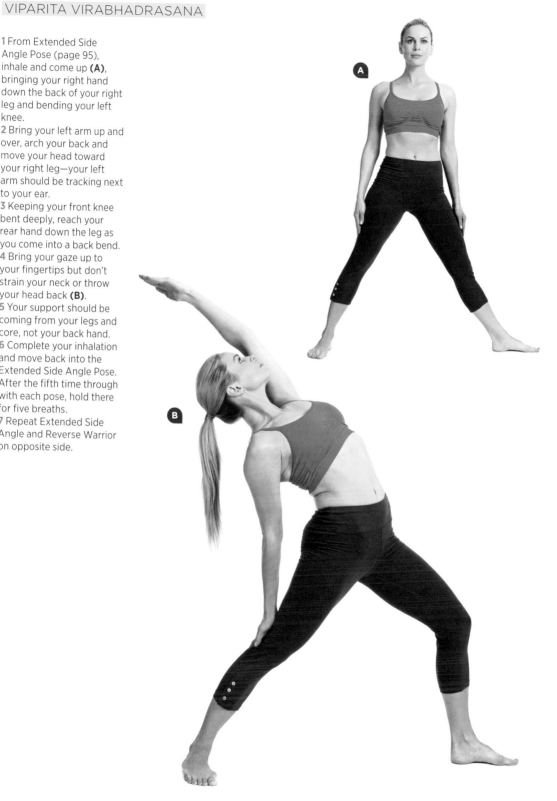

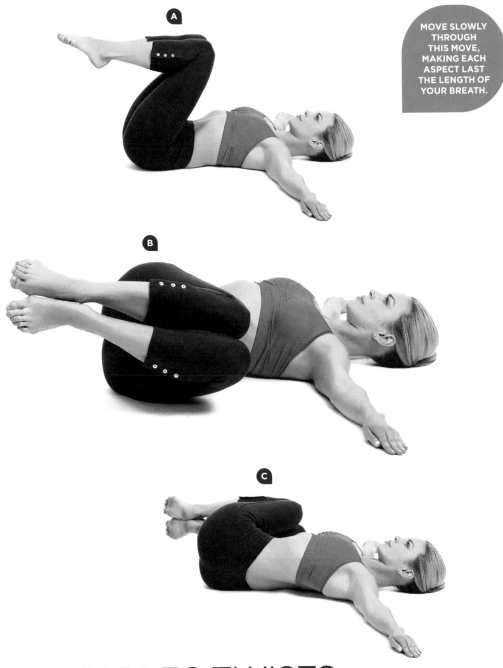

BENT-LEG TWISTS

1 Lie on the floor, knees bent 45 degrees in toward you, feet off the floor and your arms outstretched on the floor **(A)**.
2 Inhale, and keeping your legs and knees together, drop both legs to the left. Don't let your knees or legs touch the floor, and come as low as you can without your back arching or holding your breath **(B)**.
3 Exhale and lift legs back up and over to the right **(C)**.
4 Keep your lower back gently pressed into the floor and squeeze your navel inward, to ensure your core is working.
5 Repeat five times on each side. Rest and repeat.

VARIATION Squeeze a cushion or block between your inner thighs to make this move more challenging.

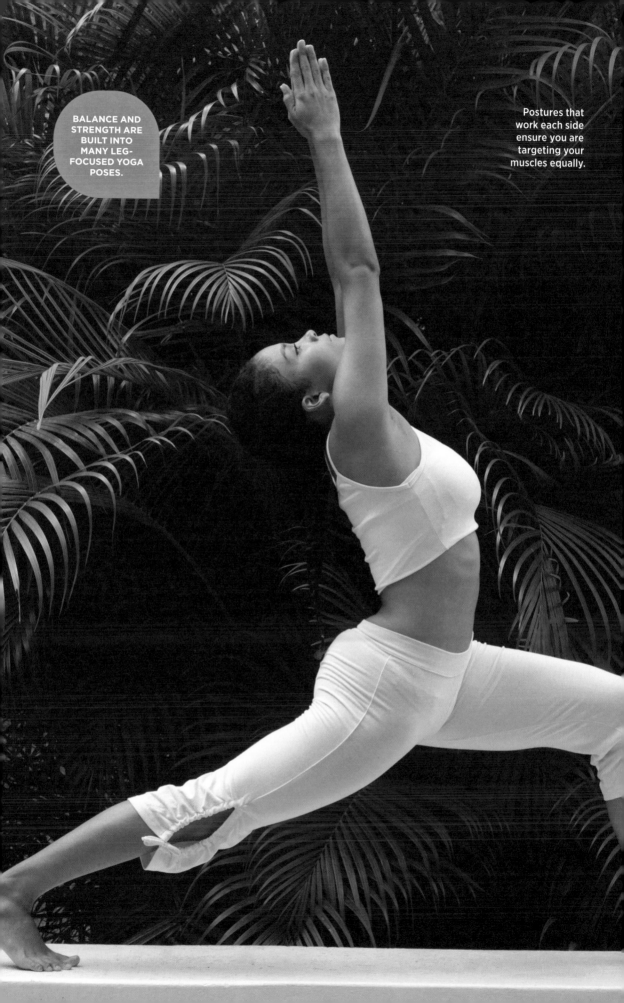

BALANCE AND STRENGTH ARE BUILT INTO MANY LEG-FOCUSED YOGA POSES.

Postures that work each side ensure you are targeting your muscles equally.

SCULPT STRONG, LEAN LEGS

FIRM UP THE QUADRICEPS, HAMSTRINGS AND CALVES WITH POSES THAT BUILD STRENGTH AND FLEXIBILITY WHILE MOVING THROUGH A FULL RANGE OF MOTION.

Look at people who practice yoga regularly and you'll notice most have lean, strong hamstrings and quadriceps muscles. These are among the biggest muscles in your body, and strengthening them means your body's fat-burning power—even at rest—will shoot up, helping boost the body's natural calorie-burning engine. This workout is designed to combine muscle strengthening with flexibility, giving you a well-rounded workout that not only gets you stronger but also increases the range of motion in your joints, reducing your risk of injury that can occur with age or activity.

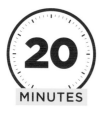

HOW TO DO IT

BUILD LEG STRENGTH

Get strong and shapely thighs and calves with these poses, which use your own body weight for resistance while also increasing flexibility. Follow the poses in order, and modify some of the more challenging parts of this to suit your fitness level. Do it twice if time permits.

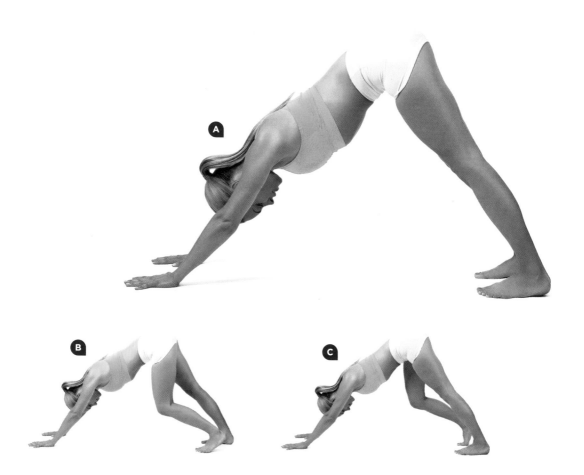

DOWNWARD-FACING DOG

ADHO MUKHA SVANASANA

1 Kneel on all fours, legs hip-width apart, hands under your shoulders and fingers fanning out **(not shown)**.
2 Exhale and curl your toes under, straighten your arms to lift your upper body and extend your legs to lift your hips toward the ceiling **(A)**.

3 Press your shoulder blades back and relax your head. Draw in your abs, pull up your thigh muscles, press your thighbones back and imagine your heels stretching back **(B)**.
4 Straighten legs (or keep knees slightly bent). Point your tailbone to the ceiling

and heels toward the floor. Focus on lengthening the legs and lifting the tailbone.
5 To help warm your legs at the start of your practice, alternate bending and straightening each leg up to 10 times **(C)**.
6 Take five deep breaths, rooting hands into the floor

and keeping thigh muscles strong and head relaxed.
7 To exit, bend knees and return to all fours. Repeat.
8 For extra toning, squeeze a block or cushion between your thighs.

CHAIR POSE

UTKATASANA

1 Stand tall with feet hip-distance apart, and squeeze the thin side of a block (or use a small cushion) between your thighs.
2 Inhale and lift your arms over your head, palms facing inward **(A)**.
3 As you exhale, bend your knees and lower your hips as if you're sitting down on an imaginary chair, squeezing the block between your thighs until they are almost parallel to the floor **(B)**.
4 Don't let your knees project over your toes. As you look down, you should be able to see your big toes.
5 Look straight ahead, relax your shoulders and take five breaths, sinking a little deeper in with each exhalation and lengthening your torso on each inhalation.
6 Keep your tailbone pointing down and ensure your abdomen is engaged—don't concave your back and keep your spine straight.
7 Straighten your legs to come up. Repeat three times.

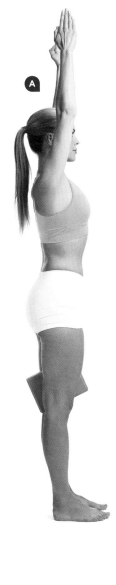

A

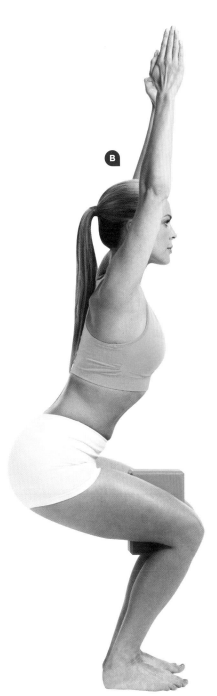

B

FOR A CHALLENGE, MAKE THE SQUAT EVEN DEEPER, BUT KEEP KNEES BEHIND TOES.

PLANK POSE WITH MOUNTAIN CLIMBERS

1 Start on all fours, hands shoulder-width apart directly under shoulders **(not shown)**.
2 Inhale, tuck your toes under and straighten legs so you're in a diagonal line from head to feet.
3 Exhale and tuck in chin, keeping the back of your neck long, forming a line from head to spine **(A)**.
4 Engage your abdominals, drawing them toward your spine. Breathe evenly; don't hold your breath.
5 Round upper back and spread shoulder blades apart to broaden your back.
6 Root your palms into the floor with your fingers fanning out, elbows straight but not locked.
7 Engaging your belly and keeping your Plank steady, bring your right knee up toward your right elbow. Bring your knee as high as you can while engaging your core **(B)**.
8 Repeat with your left side, bending and bringing your left knee to your left elbow.
9 Do 20 altogether, 10 on each side. Beginners start with five on each side and build up. Rest and repeat.

KEEP YOUR PLANK AS STRAIGHT AND FIRM AS YOU CAN AS YOU LIFT EACH LEG.

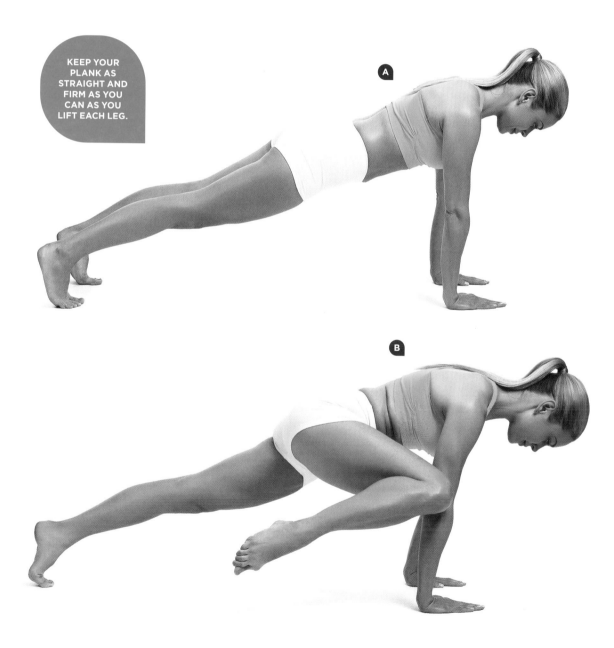

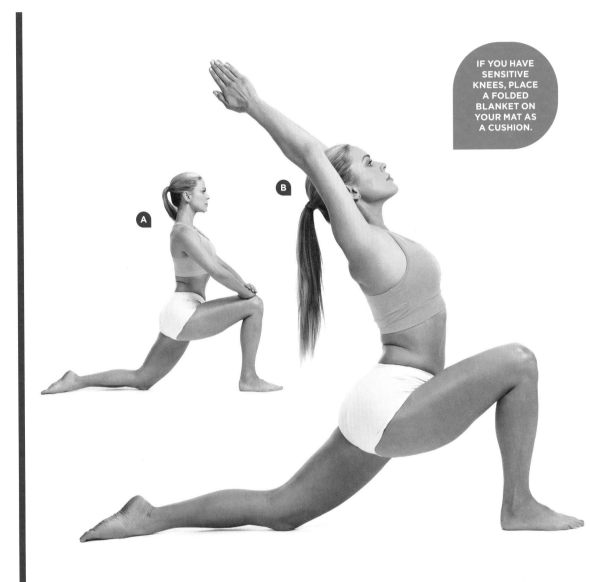

CRESCENT MOON POSE

ANJANEYASANA

1 Stand with legs about hip-distance apart, arms at sides. Inhale and step your left leg back, placing the top of your foot and knee on the floor and resting hands on right knee **(A)**.

2 Exhale. Lift arms up overhead, palms together. Open your chest, drawing your hips and pelvis down and forward and root the foot of your right leg into the mat for support **(B)**.

3 Draw in your abdominals. Keep your shoulders down and relaxed and draw your shoulder blades together.

4 Lengthen your neck while continuing to gaze forward.

5 Take three to five breaths, then straighten back leg off the floor **(not shown)**. Stay here for another three to five breaths. Repeat.

6 To exit, exhale, bring your hands to the floor, step your left foot back to the right one and slowly come up. Switch sides and repeat.

KEEP YOUR KNEE BENT 90 DEGREES, AND ALIGNED OVER THE ANKLE.

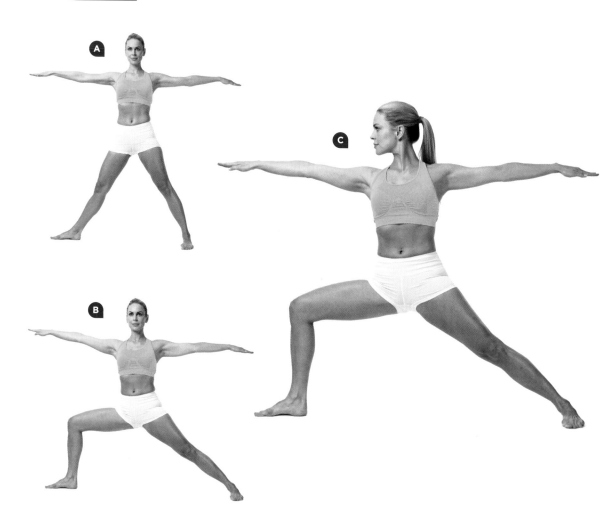

WARRIOR II

VIRABHADRASANA II

1 Stand with feet together, arms at sides. Step left foot back, turning right foot to face forward and left foot in about 15 degrees, so right ankle points to the arch of the left foot.

2 Inhale and extend arms out from shoulders, parallel with the floor, palms facing down. Lengthen arms by extending through fingers, shoulders soft **(A)**.

3 On an exhalation, bend right knee 90 degrees, shin perpendicular to the floor **(B)**. Lift your inner arches, root down the outer edges of your feet and pull up the thigh muscle in your back leg for stability.

4 Keeping torso facing forward, turn head to gaze over right arm, focusing on the middle finger of right hand. Inhale, straighten right leg, exhale and bend it three times to 90 degrees, then lower into the pose and hold for five breaths **(C)**.

5 Your torso should rise from your hips and your arms should feel as if they're being stretched in opposite directions.

6 Repeat on the other side.

WIDE-LEGGED FORWARD BEND

PRASARITA PADOTTANASANA

1 Step feet about one-and-a-half leg-length's distance apart with your feet parallel and hands on your hips **(A)**.
2 Lift your inner arches and press the outer edges of your feet to the floor.
3 Contract your thigh muscles without locking your knees. Drawing your tailbone down, lengthen your spine and open your chest to the ceiling. Look up without straining your neck.
4 Keeping your legs strong, hinge forward from hips and bring hands or fingertips to the floor or put your hands on your thighs.
5 Draw your tailbone up toward the ceiling. Inhale, straighten your arms and look forward **(B)**. Take five deep breaths, keeping your spine long and letting your head relax down.
6 Bring the crown of your head to the floor (or as low as it will go) and hold for three to five breaths **(C)**. Rest your head on a block if needed (see Variation).
7 To exit, exhale and bring your hands to your hip joints.
8 Inhale, press your feet into the floor, contract your tummy and come up.

CONTRACT YOUR QUADS TO BUILD STRENGTH WHILE RELEASING THE HAMSTRINGS.

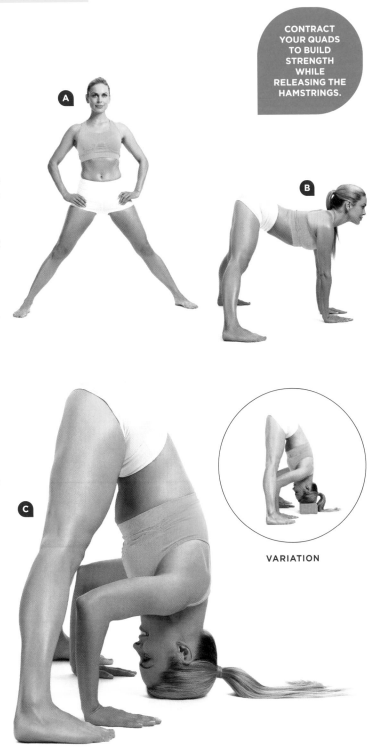

VARIATION

ONE LEG BENT SEATED EXTENSION

MARICHYASANA

1 Begin by sitting with your legs straight out in front of you **(not shown)**.

2 Bend your right knee and place your foot flat on the floor with a few inches between it and your inner thigh or knee. Bring your foot only as far as it will come while your upper body remains upright.

3 Inhale and lift your right arm straight up **(A)**.

4 Exhale, hinge forward from your hips, reaching your right arm forward, rotating it inwardly. At the same time bring your torso forward.

5 Bring the back of your arm around your bent knee and your torso further forward, looking forward with your face toward your toes.

6 On an exhalation, bring your right arm behind your back to take hold of your left hand (intermediate only) **(B)** or a strap (see Variation).

7 Hold the posture for five breaths. With each inhalation, lengthen your torso and with each exhalation, come forward a little further **(C)**. Release and repeat on the other side.

VARIATION If you're a beginner or intermediate and can't join your hands in this posture, begin with a strap in your left hand. When you bring your right hand to meet it, take the strap instead, wherever it feels comfortable.

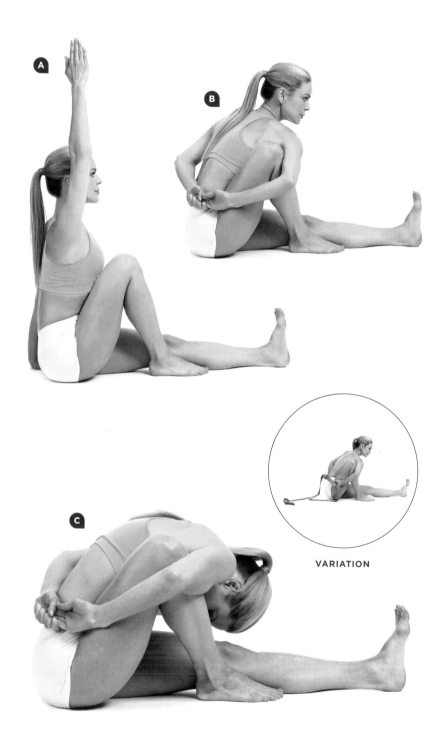

VARIATION

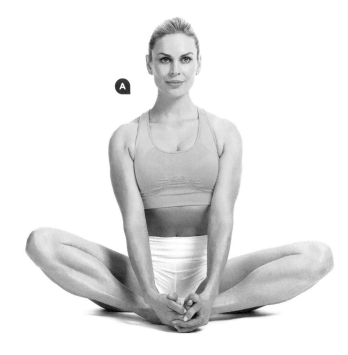

A

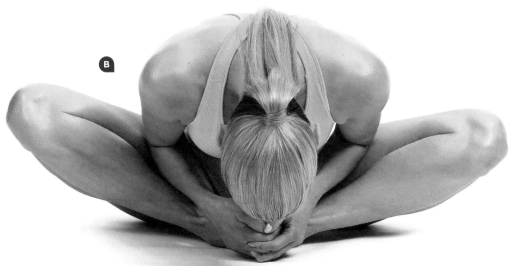

B

COBBLER'S POSE

BADDHA KONASANA

1 Sit, exhale, bend knees and draw feet together toward your groin as close to your pelvis as is comfortable.
2 Inhale and hold your feet, ankles or shins with your hands, then lengthen the crown of your head upward. Hold for five to 10 breaths (A).

3 Exhale and tilt forward from your pelvis with your spine straight—as if trying to bring your navel to your feet. Continue to inhale and lengthen spine, then exhale and tilt forward from hips as far as is comfortable (B). Take five to 10 breaths and release.

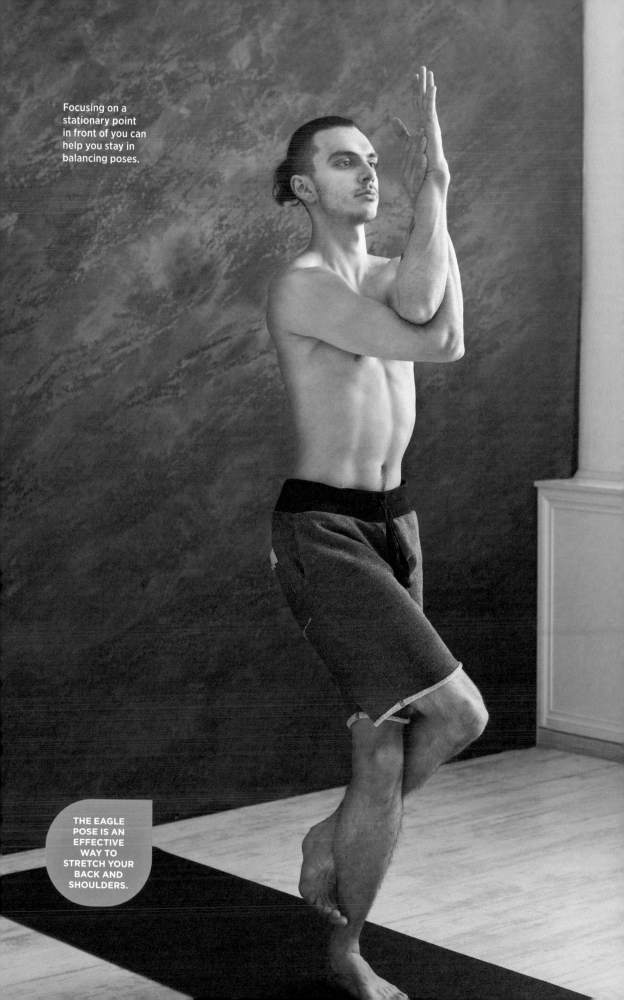

Focusing on a stationary point in front of you can help you stay in balancing poses.

THE EAGLE POSE IS AN EFFECTIVE WAY TO STRETCH YOUR BACK AND SHOULDERS.

ASANAS FOR AMAZING ARMS

YOU DON'T NEED DUMBBELLS TO GET WELL-DEFINED BICEPS AND TRICEPS. THESE YOGA POSTURES WORK THE ENTIRE UPPER BODY—NO WEIGHTS REQUIRED!

Yoga conditions the entire upper body, including the arms, using just your body weight for resistance. And because you frequently stay in a pose for several breaths, you'll extend this time under tension, which works the muscles more completely. This sequence is designed to challenge your arms as well as your chest and shoulders, so you may feel a little sore after the first few times. If you have a preexisting shoulder or wrist injury, modify the moves to prevent pain. It may help to start with a few rounds of Sun Salutation (see pages 52-53) as a warm-up.

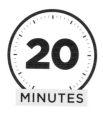

20 MINUTES

HOW TO DO IT
TONE YOUR ARMS

Time to flex! These moves are designed to work the muscles along the front and back of your arms, as well your chest, back and shoulders. Do them in the order they appear, taking time to feel your entire upper body working in balance. Repeat if time permits and modify as needed.

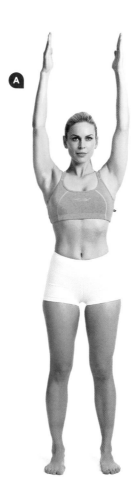

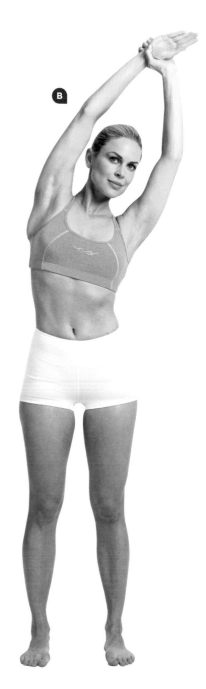

UPWARD SALUTE WITH SIDE STRETCH

URDHVA HASTASANA

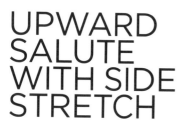

1 Stand tall with hands at sides, centering weight on all four corners of your feet, focusing on your breath **(not shown)**.
2 Turn your palms outward, inhale and lift your arms out to the side and up toward the ceiling.
3 Reach up through your hands without compressing your neck. Keep your shoulders down. Take five breaths **(A)**.

4 On an exhalation, reach both arms over to the right, feeling a stretch in the left side of your body—don't let your torso come forward. This is a side stretch so it's better to move a little to the side in the right way than a lot in the wrong way.
5 Take hold of your left wrist with your right hand. Take three breaths **(B)**.
6 Repeat on the other side.
7 Do the pose twice on each side.

EAGLE POSE

GARUDASANA

1 Stand tall with hands at sides, feet slightly apart **(not shown)**.
2 Inhale, bending both knees a little, and lift your right foot up, crossing right thigh over left and bending a little further. Point your right toes down **(A)**.
3 Exhale, lower a little further and hook your right foot over your left calf **(B)**.
4 Balance on your left leg, pressing left foot into the floor. Inhale and stretch your arms in front of you, elbows bent 90 degrees. Cross left arm over right, so left elbow is on top. Exhale.
5 Inhale and raise your forearms until you feel a stretch across your upper arms and back.
6 Bring your hands together to face each other—they may not reach, which is fine **(C)**.
7 Take five breaths here. On each inhalation, press palms together and lift elbows up a little more. On each exhalation, bend knees a fraction further, as if sitting into an imaginary chair. Repeat on other side.
8 To help you balance, focus on a point directly in front of you rather than on the floor, breathing evenly.

FOCUS ON DISTRIBUTING WEIGHT ON ALL FOUR CORNERS OF THE FOOT OF YOUR STANDING LEG.

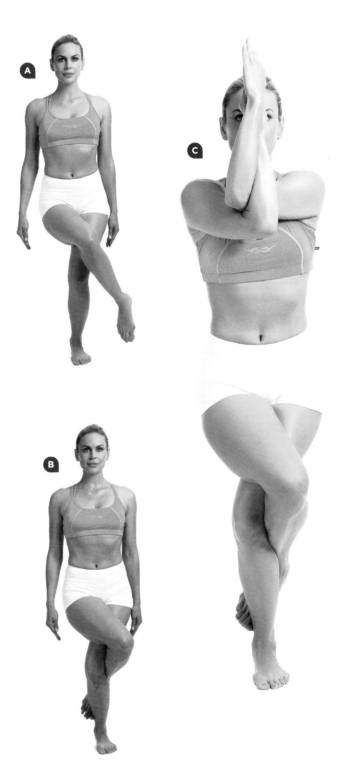

111

DOWNWARD-FACING DOG WITH ARM HOLDING OPPOSITE LEG

1 Kneel on all fours, legs hip-width apart and hands under shoulders **(not shown)**.

2 Exhale and curl your toes under, straighten your arms to lift your hips and extend your legs, raising hips toward the ceiling.

3 Draw your shoulder blades back and relax your head between your arms.

4 Draw in your abdominals, engaging your thigh muscles.

5 If you can, straighten your legs—if your hamstrings are tight, keep your knees bent. Point your tailbone to the ceiling **(A)**.

6 On an inhalation, take your left hand under your body and put it on the outside edge of your right ankle, twisting your torso to the right.

7 Look under your right arm to the ceiling, facing up. Use your left hand as a lever, helping to release and stretch your right shoulder **(B)**.

8 Take five deep breaths, drawing the ankles toward the back of the room, keeping your thigh muscles strong. With each exhalation, twist your body further, looking up without straining your neck.

9 Repeat on the other side.

10 To exit, come back to Downward-Facing Dog, bend your knees and return to all fours.

VARIATION If you can't reach your ankle with your hand, wrap a scarf or strap around the ankle and take hold of it with your hand.

THIS IS A DEMANDING POSE, SO IF YOU GET TIRED, COME DOWN TO YOUR KNEES.

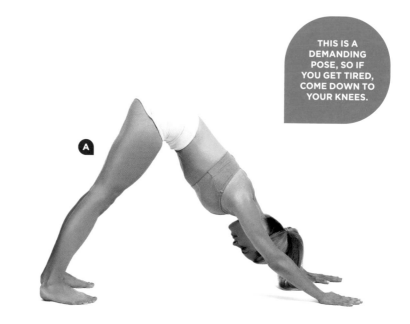

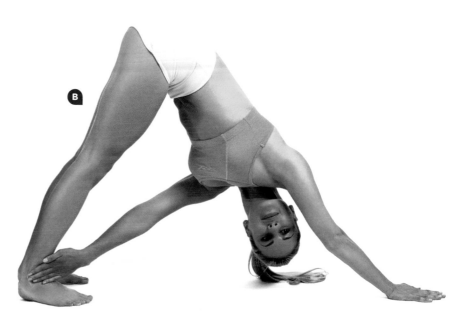

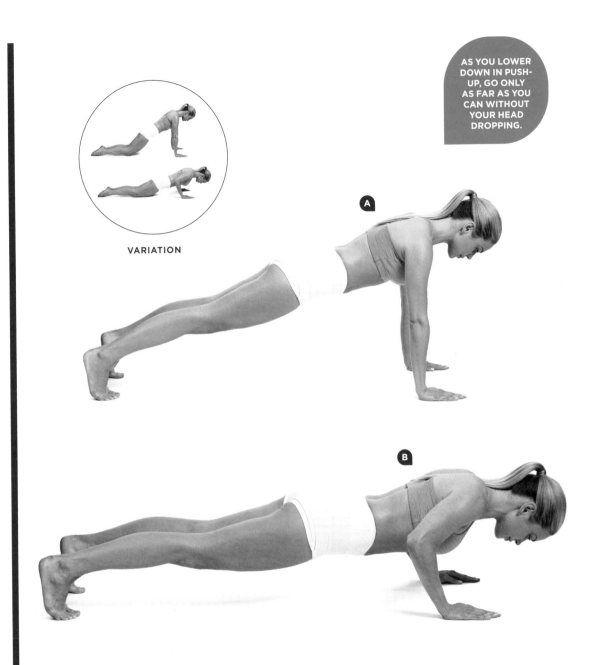

AS YOU LOWER DOWN IN PUSH-UP, GO ONLY AS FAR AS YOU CAN WITHOUT YOUR HEAD DROPPING.

VARIATION

PLANK TO PUSH-UP

1 Start on all fours with your hands slightly wider than shoulder-width apart.
2 Inhale, tuck toes under and straighten legs to form one line from head to heels.
3 Exhale and tuck your chin in slightly. Keep the back of your neck long and make a line from your head to your spine **(A)**.

4 Engage your abdominal muscles, drawing them toward your spine. Keep breathing even and long—it's tempting to hold it!
5 On an exhalation, maintaining the shape of the Plank and keeping your abdominal muscles tight, bend your arms and lower your body down **(B)**.

6 Inhale and come back up to Plank. Hold for one breath, and then lower back into the push-up.
7 Complete 10 reps. Rest for a moment and repeat.

VARIATION To make it easier, keep knees bent on the floor for the push-up, then straighten into Plank.

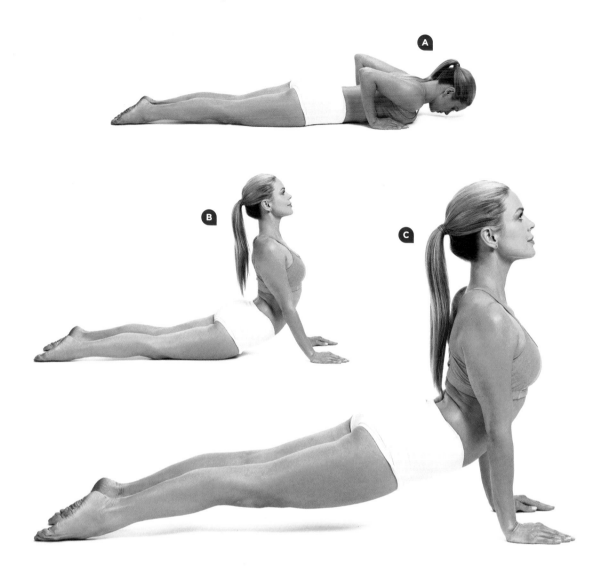

UPWARD-FACING DOG (COBRA VARIATION)

URDHVA MUKHA SVANASANA

1 Lie facedown on the floor, with the tops of your feet and palms on the floor and elbows bent and close to sides **(A)**.
2 Inhale, keeping your head in line with your spine, pressing your palms into the floor as you lift your chest and torso slightly off the floor.
3 Using your hands, feet and rising body for momentum, exhale and slide your hips forward.
4 Inhale, lifting your torso up off the floor so your chest opens and points upward, and straighten your arms **(B)**.

5 Keep your legs active by squeezing your upper thigh muscles together to lift your knees off the floor while keeping bodyweight on your feet and palms **(C)**.
6 Roll the shoulders down and back, keeping your chest lifted. Lift your hips up toward your hands to help open your torso. Look forward and take five long, slow breaths.
7 To exit, roll back over your toes with an exhalation, lifting your hips into Downward-Facing Dog.

DOWNWARD-FACING DOG

ADHO MUKHA SVANASANA

1 Kneel on all fours, legs hip-width apart, hands under your shoulders and fingers fanning out.

2 Exhale and curl your toes under, straighten your arms to lift your upper body and extend your legs to lift your hips up toward the ceiling.

3 Draw your shoulder blades back and relax your head.

4 Draw in your abdominals, pull up your thigh muscles, press your thighbones back and imagine your heels stretching toward the back of the room.

5 If you can, straighten your legs; if your hamstrings are tight, keep knees slightly bent. Point your tailbone to the ceiling.

6 Lower your heels toward the floor. Don't worry if they don't touch down—rather, focus on lengthening your legs while also lifting your tailbone.

7 Take five deep breaths, keeping your thigh muscles strong and your head and neck relaxed.

8 Come back to all fours for a couple of breaths.

9 Repeat.

10 Repeat moves Plank to Push-up, Upward-Facing Dog and Downward-Facing Dog as a sequence.

BRING YOUR FEET FURTHER FORWARD IF YOU WANT TO MAKE THIS A LITTLE EASIER.

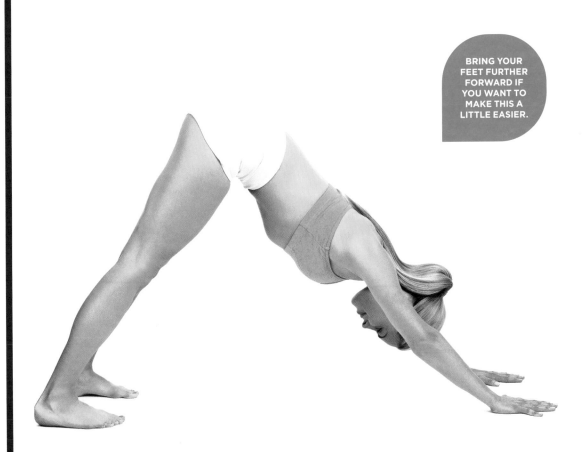

CAMEL POSE

USTRASANA

1 Kneel upright on the mat, thighs hip-width apart, and the tops of your feet against the mat **(A)**.
2 Inhale, lift your chest and torso. Keeping your hips lifted, stretch your right arm back behind you to rest on your right ankle. Exhale **(B)**.
3 Inhale and do the same with the left hand. Keep looking straight ahead with your neck straight.
4 Exhale and open your chest and shoulders, lifting your sternum gently upward.
5 Keep your neck long, chin tucked in and look forward.
6 Draw your tailbone under and your pubic bone upward to release the stretch in your quadriceps **(C)**.
7 Take three to five deep breaths, feeling the opening across your chest and hip flexors. To release, exhale into a kneeling position.
8 Repeat.

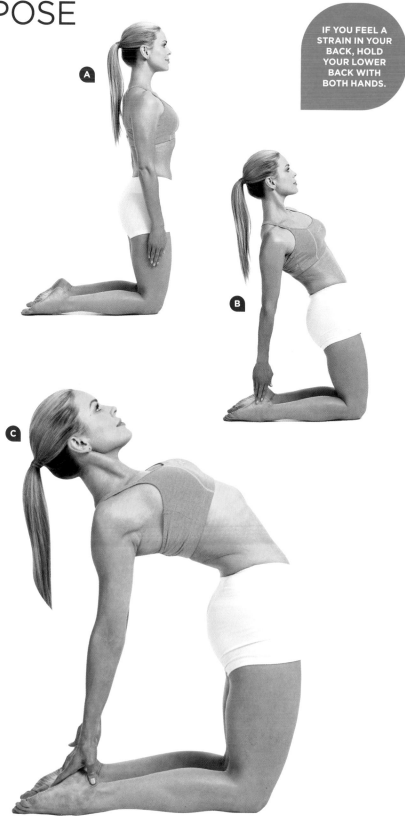

IF YOU FEEL A STRAIN IN YOUR BACK, HOLD YOUR LOWER BACK WITH BOTH HANDS.

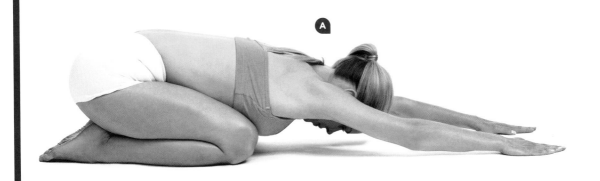

FOR A DEEPER HIP OPENING, PLACE KNEES FURTHER APART, KEEPING YOUR BIG TOES TOUCHING.

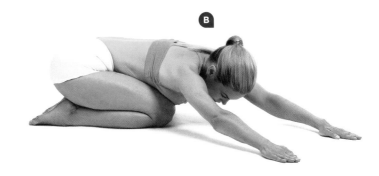

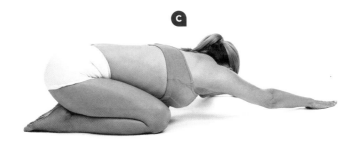

CHILD'S POSE

BALASANA

1 Kneel with knees apart, legs tucked under, pelvis resting on your shins and the tops of your feet on the floor (**not shown**). Inhale.
2 Exhale and bring arms out in front of you with palms facing down. As you walk your arms out, your torso comes forward so it

drapes between your thighs. Relax your head and neck and feel your shoulders sink to the floor (**A**).
3 Keep arms active by pressing fingertips into the floor, feeling the stretch in your arm. Take five breaths.
4 Now move both arms out to the

right and drape your torso over your right bent knee. Feel the stretch in your left side and keep your arms active and working. Take five deep breaths (**B**). Repeat on the left side (**C**).
5 During this posture, try to increase the stretch by a fraction on each exhalation.

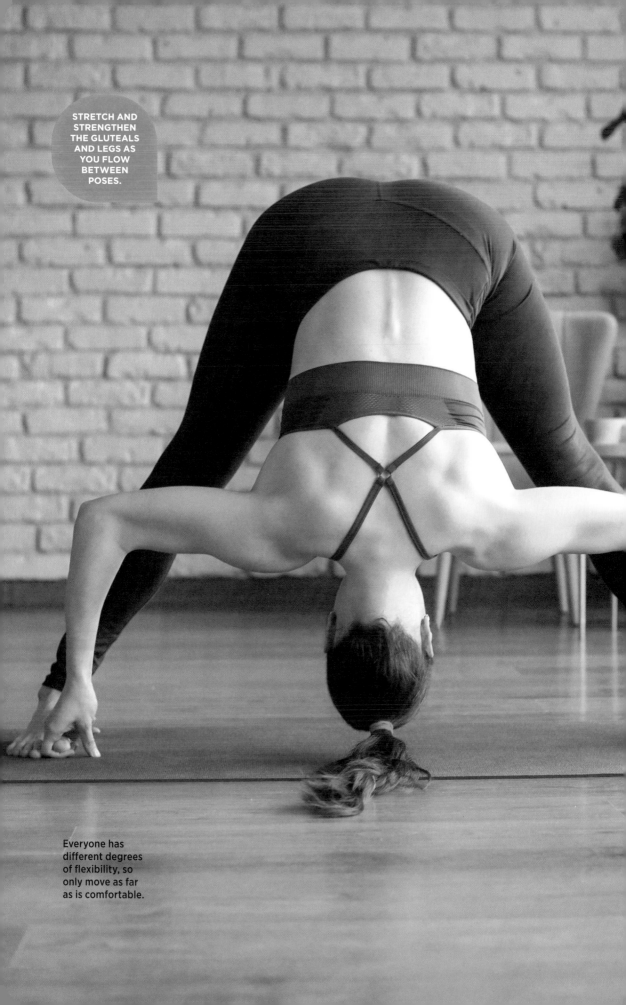

STRETCH AND
STRENGTHEN
THE GLUTEALS
AND LEGS AS
YOU FLOW
BETWEEN
POSES.

Everyone has
different degrees
of flexibility, so
only move as far
as is comfortable.

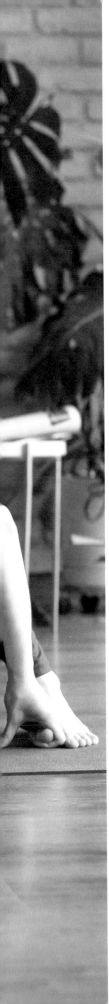

SHAPE A FIRM YOGA BUTT

ACTIVATE YOUR GLUTES AND HAMSTRINGS AND SCULPT YOUR BOOTY WITH A SEQUENCE OF POSES THAT TARGET THE ENTIRE REAR VIEW.

Ah, the famous yoga butt! Whether they set out to achieve it or not, many seasoned yoga practitioners have admirably toned bottoms. That's because so many yoga postures work the gluteal muscles, as well as those that surround them. These are muscles that rarely get used in our sedentary lifestyles, so it's especially effective. This workout strengthens and stretches the entire lower body with poses that are repeated, so your own bodyweight is used as a force of resistance to build strength. Do the entire sequence in the order it appears to build strength while increasing flexibility.

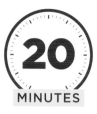

20 MINUTES

HOW TO DO IT
GET A SEXY BUTT

Strengthen and stretch your gluteals as well as your hips and legs with these flowing poses that rely on body weight for resistance. For best results, warm up with the Sun Salutation series on pages 52-53, then do the sequence in the order it appears, modifying as needed.

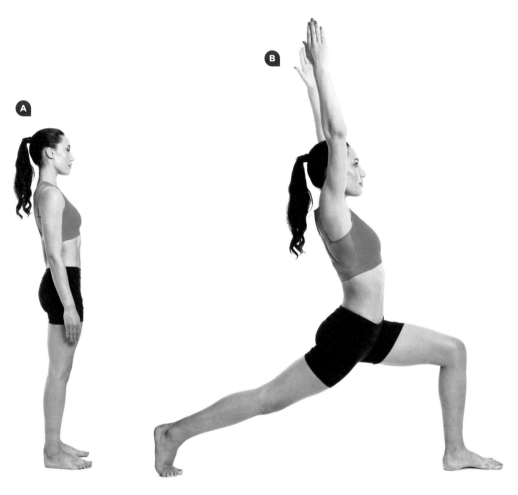

RUNNER'S LUNGE

1 Stand tall with arms at sides **(A)**. Step the right leg back one leg's-length, right toes tucked under, right ankle drawing backward.
2 Inhale and stretch arms overhead while bending the left knee until the left thigh is parallel to the floor,

balancing on the ball of the right foot.
3 Sink your hips and pelvis downward without jutting forward. Point the heel of the right foot behind you.
4 Relax the shoulders down, look straight ahead and take five breaths **(B)**.

5 Now inhale and straighten the left leg.
6 Exhale and bend the left knee 90 degrees again, lowering right knee closer to the floor.
7 Repeat eight times.
8 After the final rep, hold the pose with the left knee bent 90 degrees and right

leg straight. Lengthen the torso, extend the tailbone down and sink deeper into your lunge. Hold for six to eight breaths.
9 Press down on through the left foot to stand up. Repeat the sequence with right leg forward and left leg back.

WARRIOR I POSE

VIRABHADRASANA I

1 Stand tall with feet hip-distance apart **(A)**.
2 Inhale and step right leg back a leg-length's distance, right foot flat and turned 45 degrees, left foot facing straight ahead. Square your hips toward the front by drawing left hip back and right hip slightly forward **(B)**.
3 Inhale, raise arms overhead, arms parallel, palms facing each other.
4 Exhale and bend the left knee so it's directly over the ankle, and sink the hips down.
5 Root outer edge of right foot into floor, feeling the stretch in the inner thigh. Look straight ahead **(C)**. Hold for five to 10 deep breaths. Inhale, exhale and press down into the right foot to come up. Switch sides; do pose twice on each side.

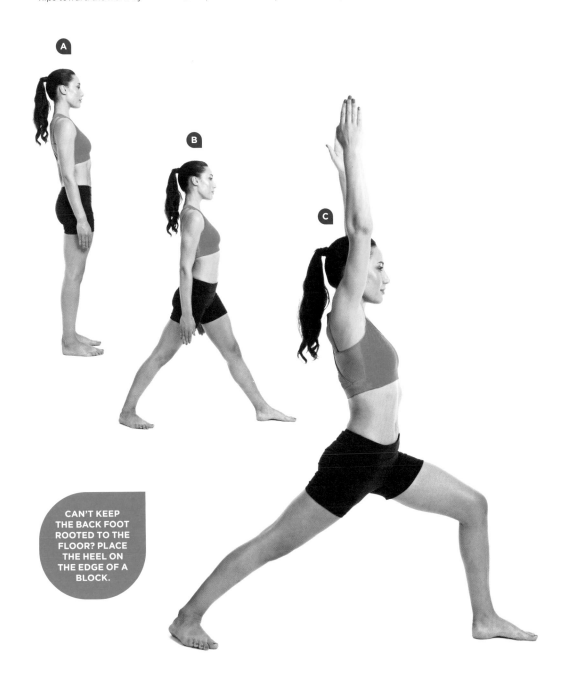

CAN'T KEEP THE BACK FOOT ROOTED TO THE FLOOR? PLACE THE HEEL ON THE EDGE OF A BLOCK.

WARRIOR II POSE

VIRABHADRASANA II

1 Stand tall with arms at sides **(A)**. Step your feet a little more than a leg's-length distance apart.
2 Turn your left foot out 90 degrees and right leg in 15 degrees so left ankle points to the arch of right foot.Keep your hips and torso facing forward.
3 Inhale and extend your arms out from the shoulders so they are parallel with the floor, palms facing down. Firm and lengthen your arms by extending through your fingers, shoulders soft **(B)**.
4 On an exhalation, bend left knee 90 degrees, shin perpendicular to the floor. Lift inner arches, root down the outer edges of both feet and pull up the thigh muscle in your right leg.
5 Keeping torso facing forward, turn your head to gaze out over your left arm, focusing on the middle finger of your left hand **(C)**.
6 Inhale, straighten your left leg, exhale and bend it five times to 90 degrees, squeezing glutes as you lower down. Then lower into the pose and hold for five breaths.
7 Repeat on the other side.

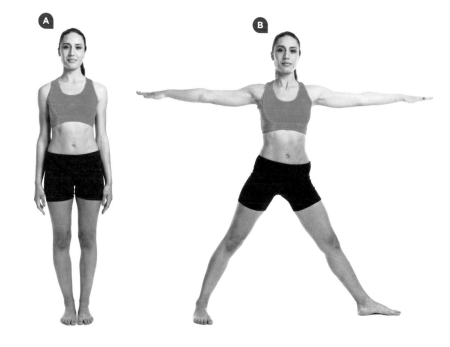

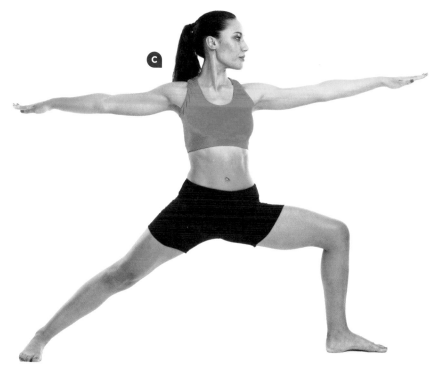

WHEN YOU LOOK OUT OVER YOUR BENT LEG, YOU SHOULD BE ABLE TO SEE YOUR TOES.

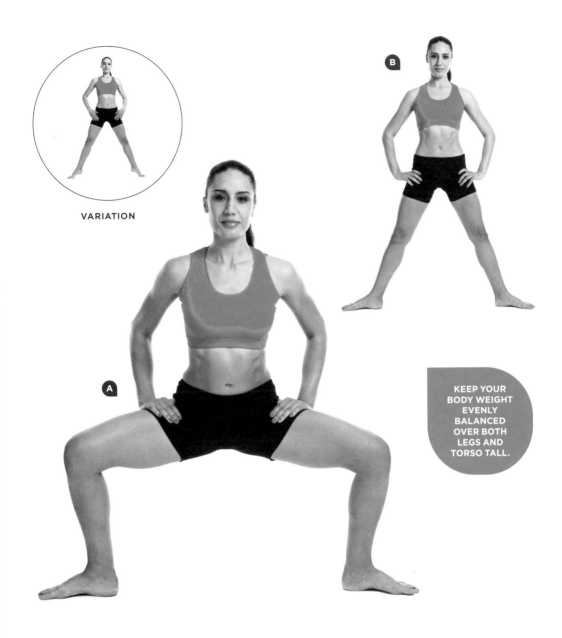

VARIATION

A

B

KEEP YOUR BODY WEIGHT EVENLY BALANCED OVER BOTH LEGS AND TORSO TALL.

HORSE-STANCE SQUATS

1 Stand with your feet about 3 feet apart and bend your knees, toes pointing out 45 degrees, hands just below your hips (A).
2 Bring hands to prayer position in front of you, or on your upper thighs—whatever feels comfortable.
3 Inhale and straighten your legs, squeezing your glutes

as you return to a standing position (B).
4 Exhale and lower back into the starting position. Continue in this way 10 times.
5 Hold pose with your knees bent and your torso straight and tall for five breaths. Straighten both legs to come up to standing position.
6 Rest. Repeat.

VARIATION For an added challenge, from the bent-knee position, gently jump up, then back into your squat. Start by doing this for every second squat and then move onto jumping with each one. If this feels like too much, lift up onto your toes—this will provide an extra workout for your calves.

INTENSE SIDE STRETCH

PARSVOTTANASANA

1 Stand tall, then step right foot forward so your feet are 3 to 4 feet apart. Turn your right foot out 90 degrees and your left foot in 45 degrees. Keep hips and torso facing right, aligning right heel with left.
2 Inhale and lift your arms up over your head. Relax your shoulders down and draw the shoulder blades together **(A)**.
3 Firm both legs, rooting your feet to the floor and lifting your inner arches.
4 Exhale and, bending from the hips while keeping them level, extend your torso out over your right leg **(B)**.
5 Place hands on floor, shin or ankle—wherever it feels comfortable. Lengthen your spine and neck, draw in abdominals and look down.
6 Draw right hip back and left hip forward to deepen the hamstring and gluteal stretch. Root right big toe into mat **(C)**. Take five to 10 breaths, then inhale, press into your feet, come up and repeat on the other side. Do twice on each side.

VARIATION If you have tight hamstrings, fold forward only as far as is comfortable and put your hands on two blocks on either side of your feet.

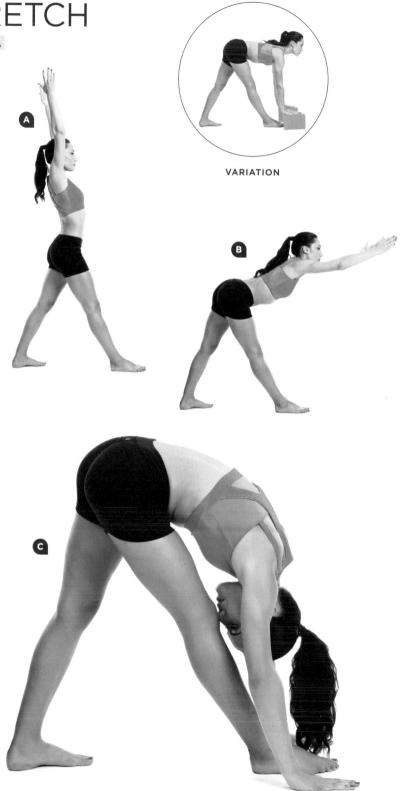

VARIATION

IF YOUR HEAD DOESN'T REACH YOUR KNEE, KEEP YOUR BACK STRAIGHT AND LOOK OUT OVER RIGHT FOOT.

REVOLVED CHAIR POSE
PARIVRTTA UTKATASANA

1 Stand tall with arms at sides **(A)**.

2 Inhale and bring your arms up over your head while bending your knees as if you're squatting to sit in an imaginary chair **(B)**.

3 Exhale and twist your torso over your thighs and to the right, bringing your left elbow over to the outside of your right thigh.

4 Bring your hands to prayer position, opening your chest. Your palms are touching and pressing into each other. Stay here for five breaths **(C)**.

5 With each exhalation, press your left elbow into your right thigh to deepen your twist and, if you feel ready, lower your butt a little further.

6 Make sure the twist is coming from your navel, not your upper back. As you twist, keep your spine extended.

7 To exit the pose, inhale and come back to the Chair Pose and exhale to standing. Repeat on the other side. Do twice on each side.

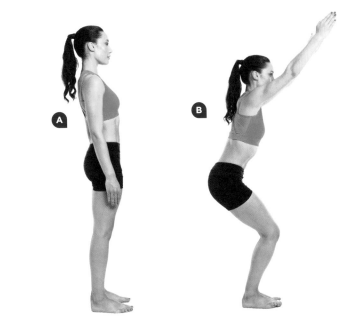

AS YOU TWIST, KEEP KNEES SIDE BY SIDE BY PRESSING FEET INTO THE FLOOR AND FIRMING THE THIGHS.

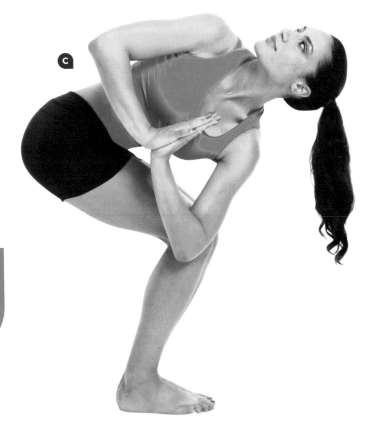

TO KEEP YOUR INNER THIGHS WORKING, PLACE A BRICK OR THICK BOOK BETWEEN YOUR KNEES.

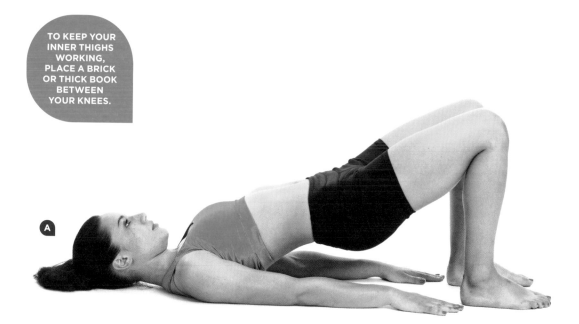

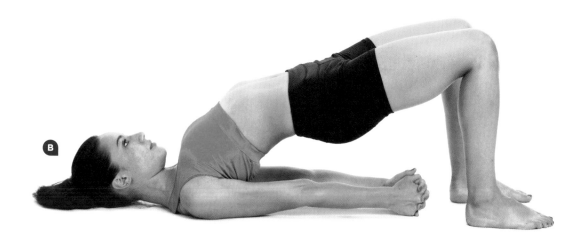

BRIDGE

SETU BANDHA SARVANGASANA

1 Lie faceup, knees bent with feet hip-width apart, thighs parallel and feet directly under your knees **(not shown)**.
2 Inhale and begin rolling your pelvis inward then upward, slowly lifting glutes and spine off the floor one vertebra at a time until your weight is resting on your shoulders. Exhale **(A)**.
3 Inhale and clasp your hands together. Breathe steadily, ensuring your thighs remain parallel, with your knees directly over your ankles—don't let your knees splay outward **(B)**.

4 Tuck your shoulders under and squeeze your shoulder blades together to further open your chest.
5 On an inhalation, press firmly into the soles of your feet and elevate your pelvis further by gently squeezing your inner thighs together. Hold for five breaths.

Do three to five sets holding each for three to five breaths. The hold is the part where you're working hardest.
6 To release, exhale and slowly roll down, beginning from your upper spine and ending in the start position.

LYING GLUTE STRETCH

1 Lie faceup on the floor with your knees bent, feet flat on the floor and hands at sides with palms down **(A)**.
2 Keep your head relaxed—if your neck is jutting back or uncomfortable, rest it on a low block or cushion.

3 Inhale and bring your right foot to rest on your left knee **(B)**. Gently press on your right knee until you feel a stretch through your outer right leg **(not shown)**. Exhale.
4 Now, inhale and clasp your hands around the back

of the left thigh (easier) or shin (more challenging). You should feel a deep stretch all the way down the outside of your right thigh and buttocks. Don't strain **(C)**.
5 Take 10 deep breaths then repeat on the other side.

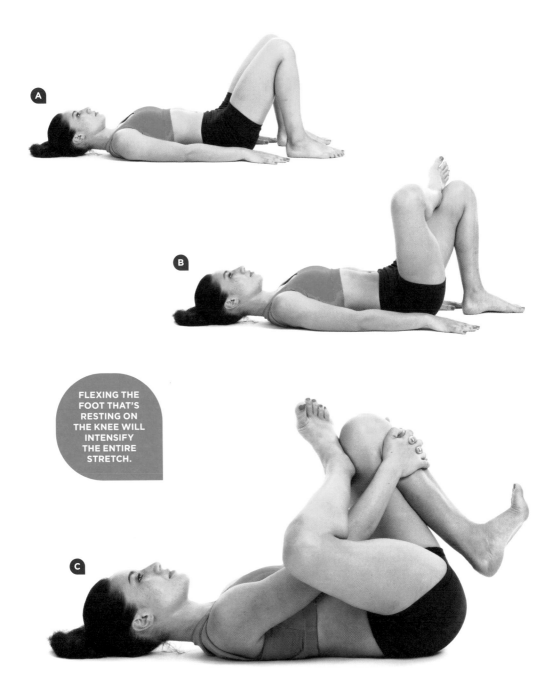

FLEXING THE FOOT THAT'S RESTING ON THE KNEE WILL INTENSIFY THE ENTIRE STRETCH.

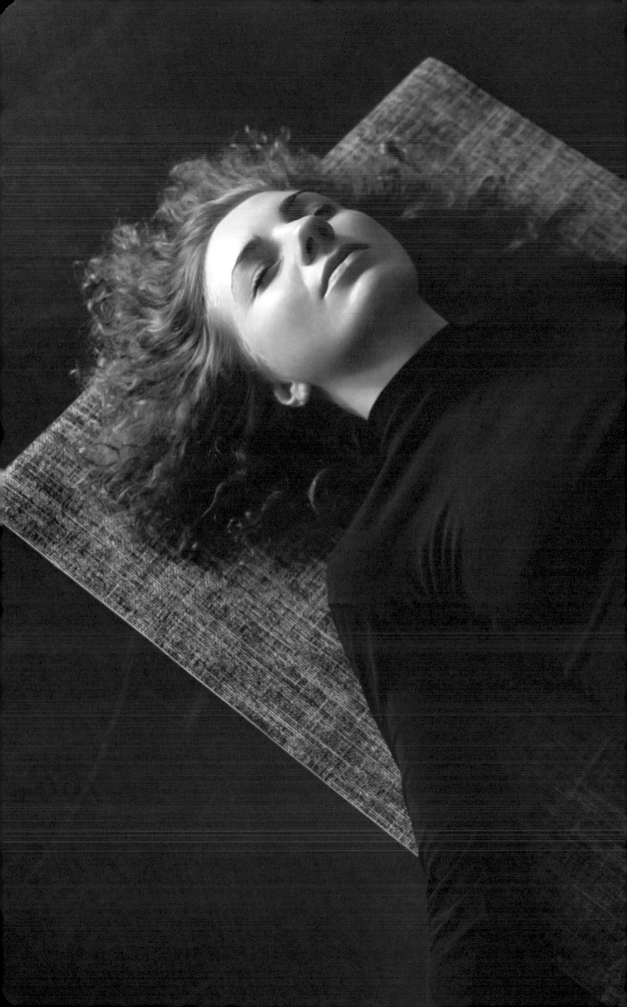

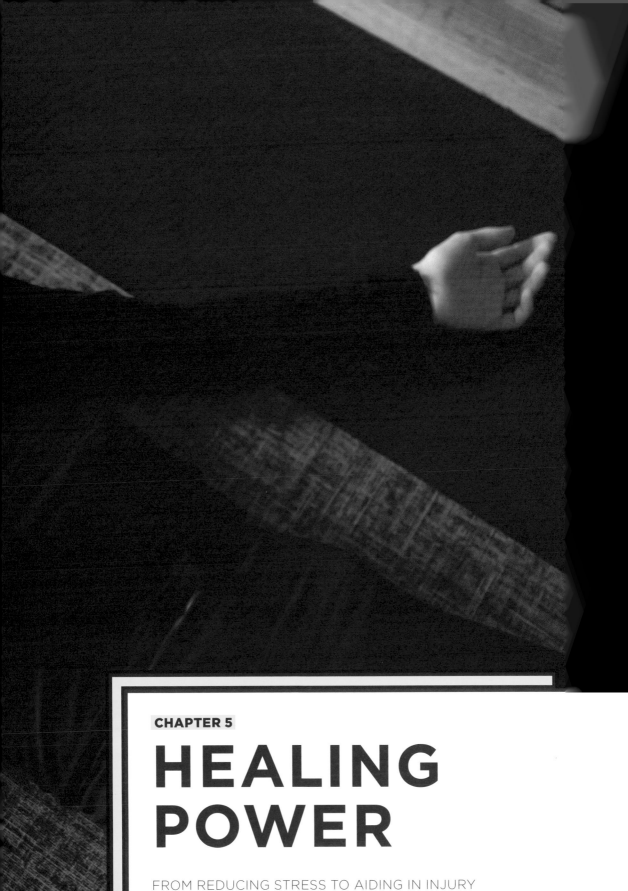

CHAPTER 5

HEALING POWER

FROM REDUCING STRESS TO AIDING IN INJURY
RECOVERY, YOGA CAN HELP YOU GET HEALTHIER.

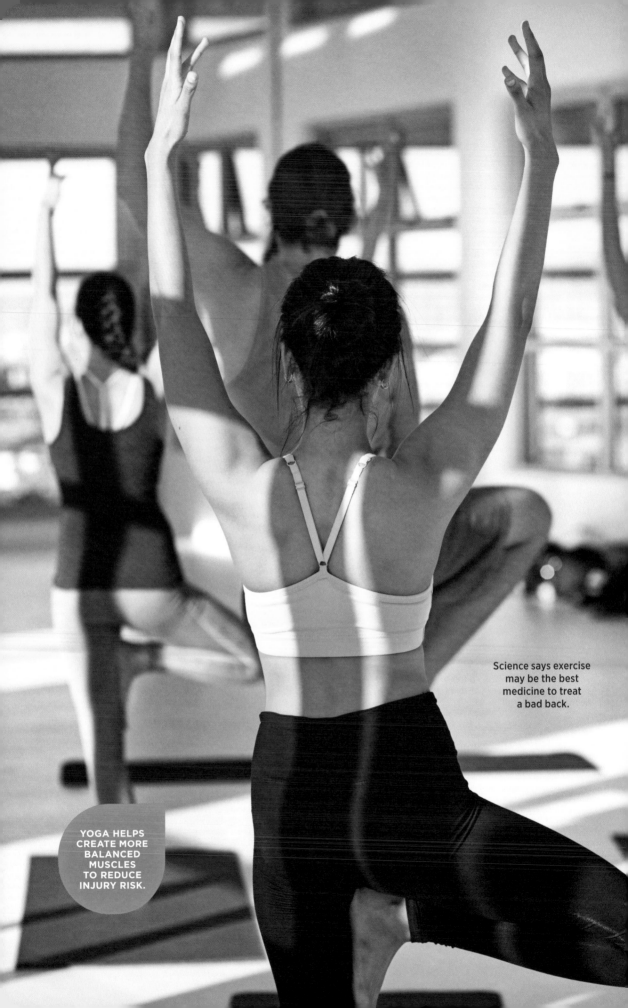

Science says exercise may be the best medicine to treat a bad back.

YOGA HELPS CREATE MORE BALANCED MUSCLES TO REDUCE INJURY RISK.

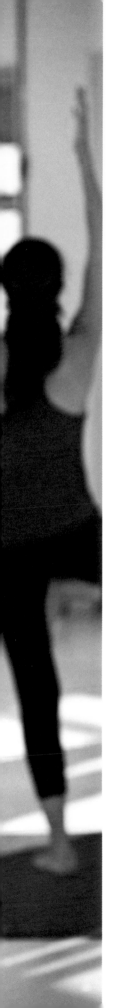

BACK TALK

YOGA CAN HELP YOU REDUCE—OR AVOID—THOSE ALL-TOO-COMMON ACHES AND PAINS IN THE BACK BY STRETCHING AND STRENGTHENING THE MUSCLES AROUND YOUR SPINE AND CORE.

Your spine is a complex structure. With 24 vertebrae (not including those in the sacrum and coccyx), 23 fluid-filled discs and a multitude of nerves, muscles and ligaments running through and attaching to it—not to mention the all-important spinal cord—there's a lot that can go wrong. Poor posture and tight, imbalanced muscles usually set the stage for aches and pain, which can be triggered by something as simple as bending over to tie your shoes. According to the National Institute of Neurological Disorders and Stroke, 80 percent of Americans will experience low back pain at some point in their adult lives and up to 70 percent of people will experience neck pain.

The American College of Physicians has endorsed new treatment guidelines for back pain that include exercise, mindfulness-based stress reduction (a type of meditation) and yoga, all of which are preferred over drugs and surgery. Movement (light exercise, gentle stretching, normal daily activities) can help loosen tight

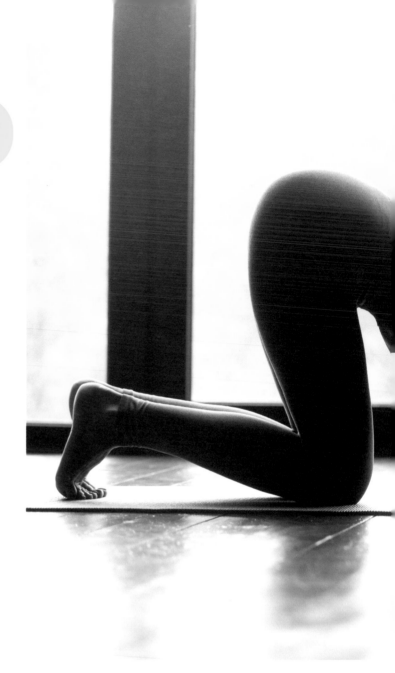

FIND FAST RELIEF.

BREATHE OUT PAIN

Three-part breathing, sometimes called "complete breath," helps release physical tension and ease aches by calming pain receptors in the brain. Here's how to try it for yourself:

Lie faceup with your back on a blanket or pillow (just enough so you're on a slight incline). Visualize your breath being directed into three areas of your torso: your belly, chest and shoulders.

Inhale, consciously filling your body from bottom to top: Inhale into the belly, then feel the breath coming into the chest and finally the shoulders.

On your exhale, consciously empty the breath from top to bottom, like you're pouring water out of a pitcher, starting with the shoulders and ending with emptying the belly.

Repeat this breathing pattern 10 times. Visualize pain leaving your body with every exhale. End with a three-minute intention: "I am open to full and complete healing. My tissues are safe and so am I."

muscles and keep circulation flowing. "Your first instinct is often not to do anything, because the muscles are in spasm and it's painful," says Nadya Swedan, MD, a physiatrist in New York City. "But it's almost always better to try to move, even if it's just to pull your knees to your chest or do a few Cat/Cow Poses." She also recommends walking, but not on the treadmill. "People tend to shorten their stride on the treadmill, or walk at an unnatural speed, or hold onto the rails, all of which can throw off your form and aggravate pain. Do it outside on flat ground," she says. (Check with your doctor first, especially if you have numbness, tingling or shooting pain or are in severe pain.)

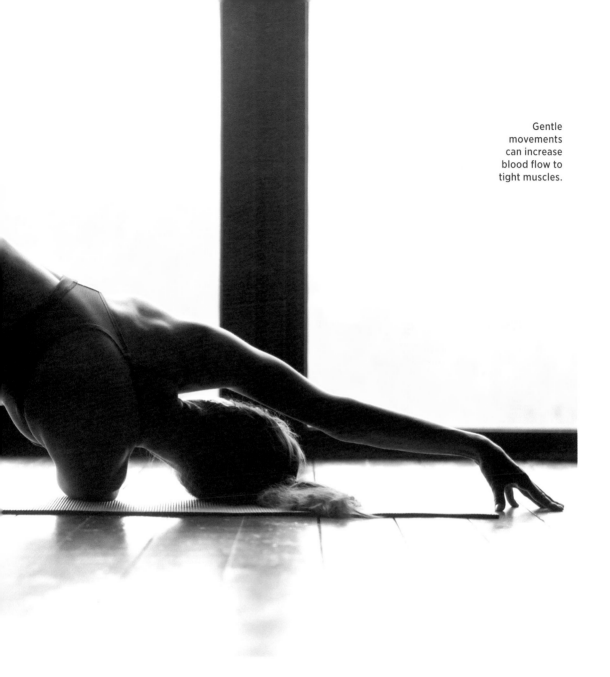

Gentle movements can increase blood flow to tight muscles.

NAME YOUR DISCOMFORT

Some backaches are caused by an irritated spinal nerve, identified as sharp, shooting, tingling and periodic pain. That happens when one of those fluid-filled discs starts protruding out (or even oozing fluid) from its space between the vertebrae, hitting a nerve. The second type of back pain is soft tissue–related, which typically feels dull and achy. Think: a sore low back after a day of skiing.

Yoga helps alleviate back pain in a few ways: Breathing practices calm the nervous system and soothe your brain's perception of pain; gentle stretches increase blood flow to injured tissues while releasing tight muscles; and strengthening poses help bolster weak postural muscles. "Yoga helps put the body in positions that require the muscles to support the skeletal system," says Erica Yeary, E-RYT, a yoga instructor and exercise physiologist in Indianapolis. "This helps re-balance the structure of the soft tissues, reduce muscular tension and improve flexibility, strength, balance and mobility."

Lisa Muehlenbein, E-RYT, a yoga teacher in Spartanburg, South Carolina, suggests restorative yoga, which lowers the body's stress response through breathing and gentle movement. If back pain is a recurring problem, "find a teacher who understands how to address dysfunction and work alongside medical professionals," she says.

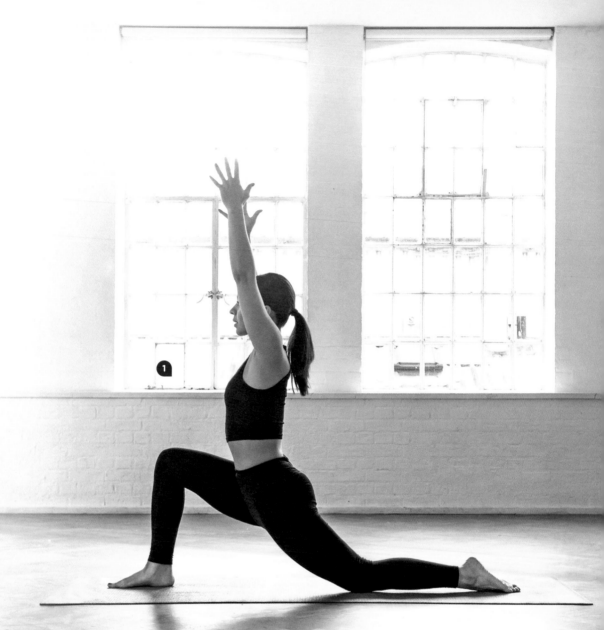

1

HOW TO DO IT

RELIEVE BACK PAIN

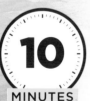

10
MINUTES

All you need for these yoga poses is a mat. If you feel pain, back off. Yoga teacher Lisa Muehlenbein uses the analogy of a stoplight with her clients. If you're feeling some stretching or strengthening, that's a "green light," and it's OK to go further. If you feel some discomfort, that's a sign to pause and reevaluate your effort, like a "yellow light." (Always make sure you're breathing.) Sharp, shooting or burning pain is a "red light," which means back off. Follow the photos to do these poses by themselves or add them to your normal practice. Check with your doctor before beginning.

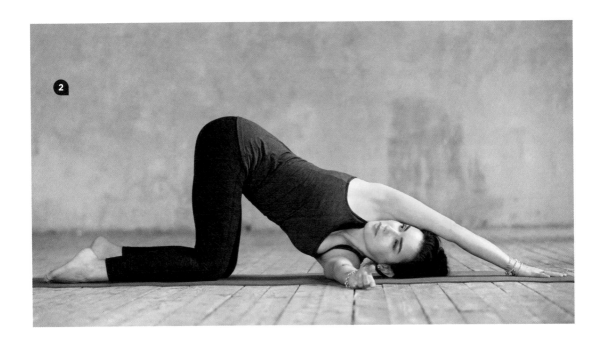

STRETCHES

1 LOW LUNGE (ANJANEYASANA)

Start on all fours and step your right foot forward, knee aligned over your ankle. Rest your hands on your front thigh or raise arms overhead, palms facing each other. Gently shift forward a few inches until you feel a stretch in the front of your left hip. Hold for 10 breaths, then switch sides and repeat. If you want to increase the stretch, lift the back knee off the floor and hold this position, breathing evenly throughout.

2 THREAD THE NEEDLE (PARSVA BALASANA)

Start on all fours, with knees hip-width apart and wrists under shoulders. Reach your left arm up to the sky, then tuck it under your body to the right. Walk your right hand forward and look to the right. Sit back slightly toward your heels. Take 10 breaths, then switch sides and repeat.

STRENGTHENERS

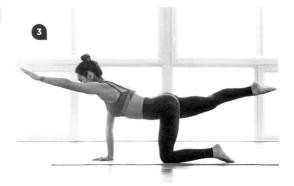

3 BALANCING TABLE (DANDAYAMNA BHARMANASANA)

Start on all fours, wrists under shoulders and knees under hips. Inhale, then exhale and extend right leg back, pressing toes into the floor. Draw your navel in and lengthen your tailbone toward your heel. Imagine a belt gently hugging around your core. Lift right foot as you reach left arm forward so it's parallel to the floor. Reach a little further as you inhale, and as you exhale, tap your right toes down. Repeat nine times, then switch sides and repeat.

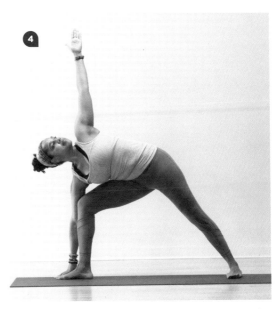

4 TRIANGLE WITH KNEE BENT (TRIKONASANA)

Stand sideways on mat with feet wide. Turn right toes toward the front of your mat and angle left toes in about 45 degrees. Extend arms and bend to right side, right knee bent. Place right hand on shin, floor or a block and reach left arm up, gazing up. Hold for 10 breaths. Stand back up to return to start; switch sides and repeat.

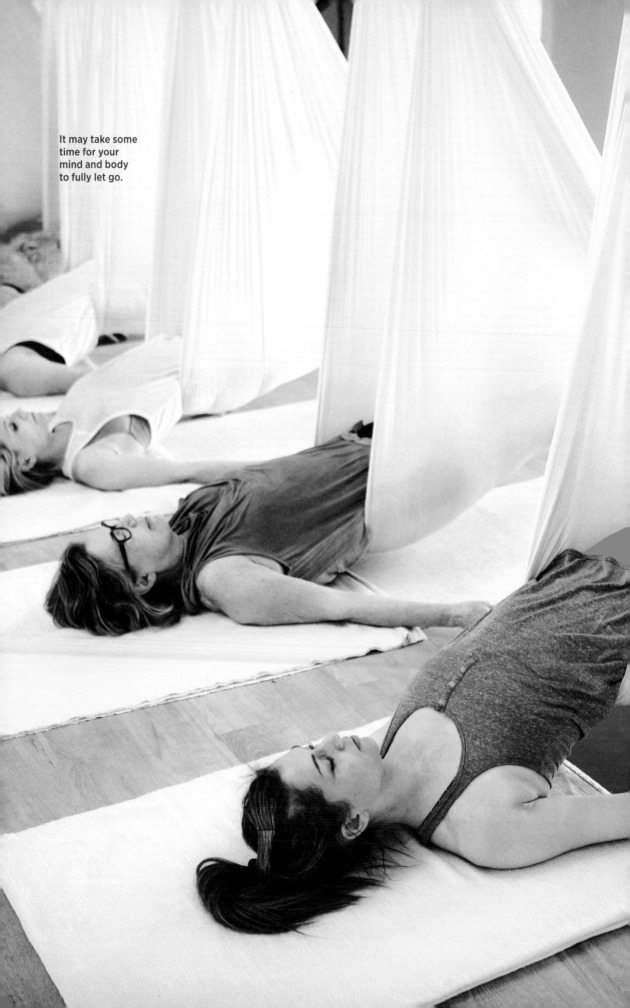

It may take some
time for your
mind and body
to fully let go.

REST, RELAX AND RECOVER

YIN YOGA COMES ON GENTLY—BUT ITS POWERFUL REJUVENATING EFFECTS WILL HAVE YOU CLAMORING FOR MORE AS YOU EXPERIENCE THE BENEFITS.

Walk into the middle of a Yin Yoga class and you might not notice much. Rather, you'd see people resting in various poses. "Yin Yoga, also known as restorative yoga, teaches your body and mind to be more mindful and to rest," says Eugene, Oregon, yoga teacher Brandy Sundberg, RYT. The practice gets its name from the Chinese concept of yin and yang: Yin is quiet, cool and calm while yang is loud, warm and dynamic—much like the world we live in.

While Yin Yoga appears serene, it's not easy. Instead of moving with every breath or holding a posture for a few breaths, you stay in a pose for at least 10 breaths or for several minutes. "You may notice that your body wants to brace itself against the stretch or that you just don't enjoy being still for that long. You have to really breathe deeply, which signals the body and brain that it's OK to rest," says Sundberg. It may not feel great at first—but stick with it and you may find a new favorite type of yoga.

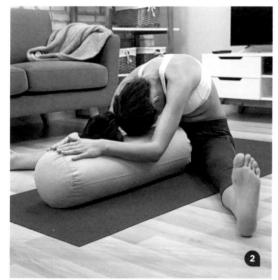

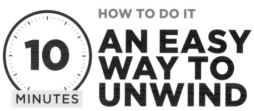

HOW TO DO IT
AN EASY WAY TO UNWIND

10 MINUTES

Try the following poses before bed or when you need to destress. If a pose starts to feel uncomfortable, bring your attention to your breath as you inhale and exhale through your nose. Hold each pose for between 10 breaths and five minutes, says teacher Brandy Sundberg. Props—bolsters, blocks, straps—are common in Yin Yoga, as they allow you to hold stretches comfortably and deepen your range of motion. You'll only need a bolster for these poses.

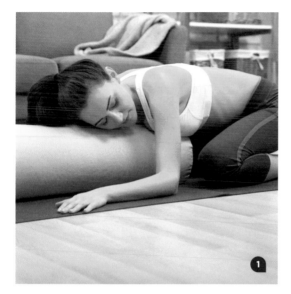

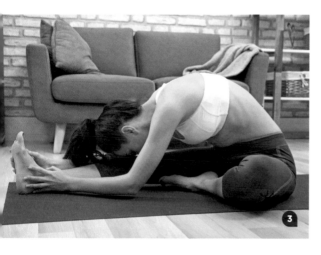

1 CHILD'S POSE (BALASANA)
Stretches the lower back
Place a bolster lengthwise on the mat in front of you. Kneel with knees hip-width apart at one end of the bolster. Rest the tops of your feet on the floor and sit back on your heels. Inhale, then exhale and round forward over your legs until your chest rests on the bolster. Place your arms on either side and turn your head to the side. (If you need extra support under your hips, place a block under you.)

2 WIDE-ANGLE SEATED FORWARD BEND (UPAVISTHA KONASANA)
Stretches the lower back and inner thighs
Sit with your legs wide out to each side, feet flexed, and place the bolster lengthwise on the mat in front of you. Sit up tall as you inhale, then exhale and bend forward from the hips (don't just round your spine). When you can't go forward anymore, round your spine over the bolster.

Rest here, placing hands lightly on the bolster.

3 HEAD-TO-KNEE FORWARD BEND (JANU SIRSASANA)
Stretches the hamstrings and lower back
Sit tall with your right leg extended in front of you and your left knee bent so the left foot rests against the inside of the right thigh. Sit tall, facing over the right leg, and inhale. As you exhale, bend forward from the hips over your right leg. When you can't go forward any further, gently round the spine over your leg. (Use a strap looped around your foot if you need to.) Rest your hands on your calf or grasp the sides of the foot. After holding, switch sides and repeat.

4 RECLINING BOUND ANGLE POSE (SUPTA BADDHA KONASANA)
Stretches the inner thighs, chest and shoulders
Place the bolster lengthwise on your mat. Sit in front of it, facing away, then gently lie back over the bolster, using your arms to guide

you (one end should be at bra-strap level or about mid-back; it might take some finessing). Exhale while bringing the soles of your feet together, letting your knees gently fall to the sides. Rest arms out to each side. (If your lower back or hips start to feel tense, place a block under each knee.)

5 RESTORATIVE BRIDGE (SETU BANDHA SARVANGASANA)
Stretches the hip flexors and quadriceps
With a bolster or block nearby, lie faceup on a mat with your knees bent and feet on the mat hip-width apart. Your heels should be aligned under your knees (shins perpendicular to the floor). Press through your heels and lift your hips to place the bolster across the width of your mat under your hips. (If you're using a block, place the wide flat part under the bony triangular structure at the bottom of your lower spine). Rest your arms out to the sides with your palms facing up. If you want more of a stretch for the hip flexors (the muscles along the front of your pelvis, which get tight and short, especially when you sit for hours a day), extend your legs on the mat.

6 CHEST OPENER IN CORPSE POSE (SAVASANA)
Stretches the chest and shoulders
Place a bolster lengthwise on your mat and sit facing away from it, legs extended in front of you. Sit up tall as you inhale, then exhale and lie back (one end of the bolster should be at around bra level or mid back). Let your arms rest out to your sides and allow your legs to relax.

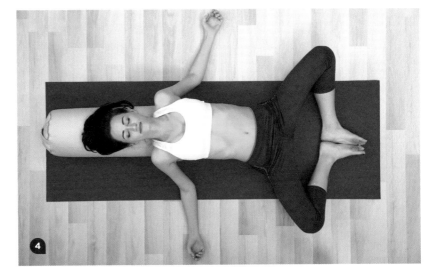

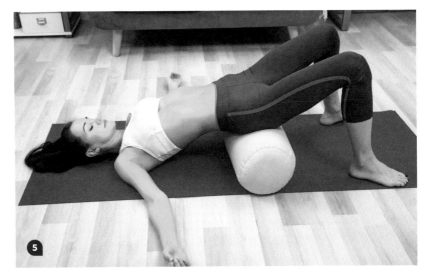

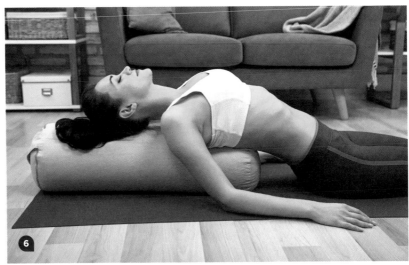

Special Thanks to Contributing Writers

Lisa Ash Drackert, Sarah Kucera, Brittany Risher

CREDITS

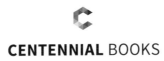

CENTENNIAL BOOKS

An Imprint of
Centennial Media, LLC
1111 Brickell Avenue, 10th Floor
Miami, FL 33131, U.S.A.

CENTENNIAL BOOKS is a trademark of Centennial Media, LLC

ISBN 978-1-951274-92-4

Distributed by
Simon & Schuster, Inc.
1230 Avenue of the Americas
New York, NY 10020, U.S.A.

For information about custom editions, special sales and premium and corporate purchases,
please contact Centennial Media at contact@centennialmedia.com.

Manufactured in China

Publishers & Co-Founders Ben Harris, Sebastian Raatz
Editorial Director Annabel Vered
Creative Director Jessica Power
Executive Editor Janet Giovanelli
Features Editor Alyssa Shaffer
Deputy Editors Ron Kelly, Anne Marie O'Connor
Managing Editor Lisa Chambers
Design Director Martin Elfers
Senior Art Director Pino Impastato
Art Directors Patrick Crowley, Jaclyn Loney, Natali Suasnavas, Joseph Ulatowski
Copy/Production Patty Carroll, Angela Taormina
Senior Photo Editor Jenny Veiga
Photo Editor Keri Pruett
Production Manager Paul Rodina
Production Assistant Alyssa Swiderski
Editorial Assistant Tiana Schippa
Sales & Marketing Jeremy Nurnberg